EDUCATION FOR NURSING

EDUCATION
FOR NURSING

A History of the University of Minnesota School

BY JAMES GRAY

UNIVERSITY OF MINNESOTA PRESS, MINNEAPOLIS

Library of Congress Catalog Card Number: 60-12546

PUBLISHED IN GREAT BRITAIN, INDIA, AND PAKISTAN BY THE OXFORD UNIVERSITY PRESS,
LONDON, BOMBAY, AND KARACHI, AND IN CANADA BY THOMAS ALLEN, LTD., TORONTO

*For help with the difficult job of securing illustrations for this
book, the publisher thanks Cecilia Hauge, Pearl McIver, Helen
Goodale Florentine, Myrtle Hogkins Coe, Lucile Petry Leone,
Rena Boyle, Dorothy Slade Kurtzman, Anna Jones Mariette,
Alice Fuller, Perrie Jones, Alma O. Scott, Maxine B. Clapp of
the University Library, the University News Service,
and the University Photo Laboratory.*

TO A FAVORITE ALUMNA
OF THE SCHOOL OF NURSING,
UNIVERSITY OF MINNESOTA,
MY NIECE,

Ruth Perin Stryker

Foreword

HERE, in this book, one gains insight into the creation of a profession — nursing. Here, too, the author highlights the vision which brought the concept of total care of the patient into focus. He tells of the pioneers in the great experiment in nursing education, a school for nursing which is an integral part of a university program. One learns from these pages that this experiment has affected every nursing program throughout the world.

This biography of a profession speaks, as well, of the vigorous and articulate leadership which developed the first true university school of nursing and the many programs basic to it. It eloquently bespeaks the endurance and persistence of dedicated women who slowly elevated the old tradition of training to the level of scientific preparation for a profession.

The medical profession, the educators, and the public all have left their imprint on the first university school of nursing. Each group has produced friends and supporters of conviction and courage equal to that of the nurses who assumed the task of conserving human life and human health through the scientific education of the student.

That financial problems have beset the school throughout its entire history, the author makes abundantly clear; that no deprivations quelled the determination to have a top-level program of education and no public pressures for more nurses altered the tenacious desire for a high quality of education for the nurse is equally clear.

"Fifty years," these pages say, "an anniversary." In fifty years the

EDUCATION FOR NURSING

School of Nursing at the University of Minnesota has made great strides: it is the first university school; it has developed scientific literacy for the nurse; it has pioneered much of the specialization in nursing; it has provided world-wide leadership; it has experimented in new programs for nursing. In fifty years curriculum-development teaching and planning has provided a corps of quality nurses whose influence has pervaded all of the continents.

As experimentation in nursing and program development was basic to the first half century of the School of Nursing, the closing pages reveal that experimentation and change will be implicit in the planning for the next fifty years. The nursing arts will continue to be refreshed by advances in science, the sociological aspects of nursing will receive increasing emphasis, and even greater strides will be made toward increasing the educational experiences for nursing.

The final chapters indicate that the University of Minnesota School of Nursing Foundation may provide one answer for a greater school of the future. During the next five or more decades it can sharpen and consolidate its role as an implementer, an evaluator of research for programs in nursing through the interest — as well as the dollars — that it can garner for the school. It is the means through which nursing and the public can collaborate in efforts to raise funds to support scholarship, to encourage new trends and developments, to strengthen the financial base, to develop community respect and understanding of need through encouragement of endowments and planned program financing.

That this book has a value for all interested in education and the professions is remarkably evident. It highlights the role of the doctor and the citizen in the development of a university school of nursing which from its very beginning practiced careful selection and required high standards of program and performance. It traces the struggles, the resistances encountered even from enlightened people, in evolving a profession from an apprenticeship system. This book should appeal to all professions, and the acceleration in momentum of a dynamic program under dynamic leadership which rolls over all impediments as it moves on should excite every reader in these days of indecision and uncertainty.

Mrs. Walter W. Walker
President, University of Minnesota
School of Nursing Foundation

Table of Contents

EDUCATION FOR NURSING

Prologue: Emergent Profession

THIS is the story of how, in the first decade of the twentieth century, a unique experiment in education was begun, fostered, and brought through all the trials of disbelief and indifference to a high level of success. The School of Nursing at the University of Minnesota was the first training center of its kind to be sponsored, anywhere in the world, by an institution of higher learning. When Dr. Richard Olding Beard and a few of his colleagues stood back and took a long, steady look at tradition centuries old and, having done so, urged the establishment of a university school of nursing, they performed a service the significance of which has come to be generally recognized. In that moment the history of the healing arts took a new turn and all subsequent developments in the delicate, complex, universally influential work of the nurse have been affected.

It would, of course, be wrong to suggest that if this lead had not come from Minnesota it might not presently have come from somewhere else. An awareness of the need for change was in the air, and the wonder of human inspiration is that it can be relied upon to give reality to vision, late or soon. Yet the fact remains that a group of people at Minnesota did show the hardihood to make a start. Within the confusion of conflicting impulses they found a new concept of responsibility and shaped it into an instrument of progress.

A backward glance through the scrapbook of the nurse's history may serve to indicate how important their decision was. Those indefatigable dramatists of human experience, writers and painters, have recorded many impressions of what her position long continued to be as age after age repeated the same anecdotes about her.

In general, practitioners of the healing arts have fared well at the hands of artists. The pathetic dependency of the sick has always made them eager to believe in the superior powers of doctor or nurse. A composite portrait of the physician, put together of the features noted usually with approval and sometimes with awe by novelist and poet, would show him as a figure characterized by poise and reserve, by strength, tolerance, and untiring devotion to duty. A famous painting of the nineteenth-century story-telling school of art presents this embodiment of the virtues of the healer as a watcher at the bedside of a sick child, oblivious of everything in the humble cottage except the approaching sign of crisis which his authority must confront and his skill control. In the arts the doctor has always worn his prestige among human types with a special benignity.

The nurse has received considerably less appreciative treatment. In one familiar literature of tenderness — that of the folk verse or song — she has been sentimentalized, as "nanny" or, worse still, as "mammy," out of all recognizability as a human being. On the other hand, a stately tradition of reverence has made the most of the nurturing aspect of the nurse's function and has raised high her symbolic status: "nurse of the arts . . . nurse of full-grown souls . . . nurse of manly sentiment." Yet, as any reasonably exploratory volume of quotations shows, there is a certain ambivalence in the poet's attitude. Phrases like "nurse of crimes," "nurse of drones," and "nurse of fools" fill out the column of references which include a surprisingly choleric one, contributed by Tennyson, to "the dirty nurse, Experience."

Unfortunately, the most vivid, full-bodied, realistic evocations of the nurse in literature are not those of the merely useful creatures of Greek drama who chattily advance the narrative and clarify the central character without developing much individuality of their own. Even the best-informed student of tradition is more likely to recall the raffish nurse of *Romeo and Juliet* whose notions of tender nurture make room for much whimsy, perversity, and even tormenting meanness. There is, most pervasive of all, the memory of that really horrible monument to the anti-heroine, Dickens' Sairey Gamp. Determined as he was to come at problems of reform by tearing away all the veils behind which society tries to hide its degradation, Dickens exposed a

4

frightening image of a shameless betrayer of faith — dirty, gin-sodden, and very nearly criminal. Unprepared for work of any kind, least of all that of the care of the helpless, Sairey Gamp presented an unforgettable image of the nurse as maker of nothing but myth and mischief. Though it was never supposed to be anything but a deliberately gross distortion of what the nurse could and should be — if only humanity would sweep out its filthy corners — the portrait of this wretched creature had hung, unchallenged as a dreadful truth, in the gallery of many a memory.

All these gestures of reverence on one side and of contempt on the other left the nurse of the nineteenth century in approximately the same position she had occupied since the beginning of civilization: that of the docile, over-worked, silent servant of the doctor. She had no prestige of her own. The virtue that was prized in her was "loyalty to the physician"; no quality more positive than that of being ready to offer an automaton's supplemental hands and feet was thought to be a virtue at all. In Europe the nurse of the period was little better than a drudge, subject to the subtly demoralizing overlordship exercised by the intellectual upon the supposedly mindless. In the United States where lines have never been so clearly defined between orders of beings, the position of the nurse was, perhaps, less humiliating. But still her lot cannot have been a happy one.

Finley Peter Dunne's "Mr. Dooley," that embodiment of the genius of common sense, probably expressed the attitude which most nearly corresponded to that of alert and responsible people. "I think," he said, "that if the Christian Scientists had more science and the doctors had more Christianity it wouldn't make any difference which ye called in — if ye had a good nurse."

The attitude toward nursing began conspicuously to change in the second half of the nineteenth century. The first person to make herself seen clearly above the crowd, as she appealed for higher standards of sanitation in the care of humanity's plagues and wounds, was Florence Nightingale. Circumstance gave her an opportunity to take a vigorous stand, and her own achievement gave her the authority to represent — almost to personify — both the responsibilities and the rights of nursing as an art. The revolution that she worked in the field hospitals during the Crimean War made her so impressive a figure among soldiers, government leaders, and all the people of England that she

5

earned brilliant prestige for herself and increased respect for her fellow workers.

It is interesting to notice that not only did she create a new design for nursing and the teaching of nursing: she herself became the archetype of nursing leader for many countries including the United States, as well as for Great Britain. All of the disciples of her cause were more than a little like her, probably, first, by native temperament, and, second, by conscious imitation.

Carefully nurtured in her father's house, well-educated by private teachers, this delicate and sensitive woman, as a young girl, conceived it her duty to seek out the sick and improve their condition. She verified and justified the nineteenth-century concept of "the new woman."

Ibsen did not write *A Doll's House* until 1879. By that time the famous "lady with the lamp" (so-called because it was her habit to make the rounds of the Crimean hospital wards after dark when the day's administrative chores had been completed) had already been spreading the light of her influence for nearly a quarter of a century. Still it remained for the playwright to present vividly the crisis in the life of the woman who wanted to be, before all else, "a human being," capable of sharing active responsibility beside the men of her life for the welfare of her family and the family of humankind.

People who like to project their imaginations far past the stated facts of the crucial situation in a work of art have spent many hours speculating about what happened to Nora, in Ibsen's play, after she slammed the door of her husband's house and went out on her own to see what "miracle" she could work upon her life. It is not at all too ingenious to suggest that she may have gone straight to work as a nurse. This was, in fact, almost the only job open, at the time, to a woman who wanted or needed independence. Further, the tragic dilemma in which Ibsen involved his character sprang out of an illness, that of her husband. In similar circumstances, prompted by the need to "help out" during family crises, many women entered service in hospitals.

The typical training school which received such women cannot have filled their imaginations with creative satisfaction. It was, in fact, not really a school at all. No one pretended that the little training they received would open a career to them. In-service instruction was offered simply to make them useful and competent servants.

For three years they lived in the hospitals under conditions which were like those of a nunnery in discipline, in isolation, in effacement of individuality. In exchange for their work student nurses received board, lodging, and instruction, plus a small monthly allowance. At the end of the training period they were free to find work where they could while a new group of girls filled up their ranks.

Actually their service was of important economic value to the hospital which returned a modicum of reward for a maximum of labor. This design continued year after year, and it was the rare woman who thought to criticize it or to dream of nursing as something that resembled a career.

Such women did, however, begin to show themselves in the late 1800's. One was Isabel Adams Hampton (later, Mrs. Hunter Robb) who entered nursing not by a kind of back door, as a means of self-support merely, but rather as though she were making a frontal attack on the portals, determined to make the hospital yield up more in the way of opportunity to service than it had ever given before.

She traveled along a route that Florence Nightingale had helped to clear of obstacles. Born in Canada and educated in much the same way that Miss Nightingale had been, she may have had the image of her famous predecessor before her when she renounced the occupation of the nice young lady of the period, which was to teach school, and went into training as a nurse at Bellevue hospital in New York. Following her graduation, she spent two years in an Italian hospital and then returned to the United States, in 1880, to become superintendent of the Illinois Training School for Nurses. This center, the first of its kind to be established beyond the Alleghenies, had a great reputation. Its tradition stood massive, formidable, and fine among the best institutions of its kind.

Miss Hampton was, by all accounts, a woman not merely of delicate breeding but one of impressive beauty and fabulous charm. Superlatives sparkle on the pages of admirers among her contemporaries who describe how they "sat on the edges of their chairs" to "drink in every word" of the eloquence she poured into her statements of mission.

A more appealing estimate comes from a pupil of the early days whose attitude is at once appreciative and critical. In this observer's view, devotion to a cause compensated in large measure for a certain meagerness in Miss Hampton's outlook. A powerful sense of direction in guiding a movement toward improvement of immediate conditions for the nurse as worker balanced a lack of genuine originality in discerning "the possibilities latent" in the art of instruction. Yet, in the end, says the analyst: "She did more to elevate the status of the nurse in this country than any person or group of persons who have followed her by her insistence upon making the position of nurses one of greater responsibility in carrying out the doctors' orders."

It was Miss Hampton, for example, who "secured authority for head nurses to write down all medical orders as directly given by attending physicians." The fact that it was necessary to make an issue of what seems now an obvious right — that of protection for the nurse against whimsicality or carelessness on the part of high authority — suggests much about the dismal level of helplessness from which the nurse had to fight her way up.

But the all important thing about Miss Hampton was her beguiling quality as personification of ardor. Even in the view of the most objective observer her look of being a kind of well-starched madonna, with "lovely coloring" and "radiant blue eyes," had irresistible attraction. The madonna's authority was at once mystic and intimately human. Trained as she was to believe in the military severity of the British system of education, Miss Hampton tried to maintain a psychological distance between herself and her students as their paths crossed in the hospital wards. But the effort was delightfully defeated daily. Trying to make an appropriate display of being the disciplinarian she would conscientiously avert her gaze from an approaching nurse. But at the actual moment of meeting she always yielded to temptation. "Cheerfulness kept breaking through," and she never failed to turn a radiant smile on her charges.

From the Illinois Training School Miss Hampton went in 1889 to the Johns Hopkins Hospital. The founder of that university had specifically instructed his trustees to establish, in connection with the hospital, a "training school for female nurses" and Miss Hampton was in a favorable position to create a superior one. That she succeeded is proved by the fact that the Johns Hopkins Hospital School of Nursing became a Mecca toward which many serious students turned their faces. Yet is was no part of Miss Hampton's plan to create a different kind of school — one that might help to lift the work of nursing to the level of a profession. The best possible standards for instruction in skills were to prevail. But the essential purpose was the old familiar one of maintaining "a continuous supply of service for the hospitals."

When Miss Hampton had been at the Johns Hopkins Hospital long enough to establish her leadership, an occasion arose for calling attention in a conspicuous way to the rights of nursing. The World's Columbian Exposition, held at Chicago in 1893, had as its theme the progress toward a new civilization made on American soil during the four hundred years since Columbus's landing. But to many thoughtful people the real significance of the Fair was that it offered a chance, not for self-congratulation, but rather to point out how much work needed still to be done.

This was particularly true of the medical profession which, just at that moment, was engaged in serious soul-searching about the standards of training. Many so-called medical schools of the nineteenth century had no real right to exist. They accepted as a student any young man who had money in his pocket with which to pay fees, regardless of the candidate's educational background or character. Year after year they turned out quacks to prey cynically on the ignorance of patients. Indeed, it was not until 1910, when Abraham Flexner made an impartial survey of conditions in medical training schools and published a devastating report, that the country was really alerted to the danger it had lethargically endured. Then, quite promptly, the "diploma factories" began to disappear.

The Columbian Exposition became a forum for speaking out the truth about the practice of medicine and about the future needs of the profession. Dr. Henry M. Hurd of Johns Hopkins was in charge of exhibits brought together by a branch of the enterprise to which the dismal and forbidding name, the International Congress of Charities, Corrections and Philanthropies, was given. (Penal institutions, universities, and hospitals were likely to find themselves placed cheek by jowl by thinkers of the time). Dr. Hurd used his opportunity to tell the accomplishments of medicine but also to define those needs to which public responsibility needed awakening.

To chairmanship of a sub-committee on nursing Dr. Hurd appointed his associate at Johns Hopkins, Miss Hampton. With spontaneous eagerness she seized the chance to be in the vanguard of a movement toward better education. Self-regulation was her theme and she lent to it all the fervor of her crusading temperament.

9

Several things happened during sessions at the fair which were to affect the future course of nursing education. Word came from half a dozen sources out of Great Britain about what its pioneers had been able to accomplish. Nurses were told, for example, that preparations had been made by Rebecca Strong of the Glasgow Infirmary to have her students admitted to Mungo's College for a short course in the medical background of nursing. This was the first time that anyone had succeeded in prying open the classroom door to let nurses in. Mrs. Bedford Fenwick of London, editor of the *British Journal of Nursing*, had come as Miss Hampton's guest to bring news of many modest steps toward an improved status for the nurse. But it was from Florence Nightingale herself — still alive and very active at seventy-odd — that the word of something like gospel came. Miss Hampton read a paper especially written for the occasion by the world's dean of nurses. In it Miss Nightingale urged that a proper training program must (1) be conducted in a well-organized hospital associated with a medical school and have a "matron" who was herself a nurse; (2) have a special organization for systematic instruction; (3) have a well-supervised residence for nurses; (4) provide for the preservation of records; (5) provide "ward sisters" (that is, head nurses) for each ward.

Renewed enthusiasm was very far from being the only result of the effort stimulated by the Exposition. At Chicago Miss Hampton suggested the desirability of organizing superintendents of nurses into a permanent body, to work for improvement in educational standards. Lavinia Dock, her close associate at the Johns Hopkins Hospital, suggested that a group made up exclusively of trained nurses could exercise vigorous moral force toward the same end. Each of these women succeeded in becoming mother to an important organization which lent both solidarity and imagination to the job of stimulating new enterprises, awakening group pride, and policing the dark corners of the nursing world. Their program had no other purpose than that of improving the nurse's ability to serve. No guild ever bespoke its faith with more zeal or with less concern for incidental matters of either financial advantage or prestige.

Miss Hampton's group, composed of administrators, was called at first the Society of Superintendents of Training Schools for Nurses. Later, with a more explicit reference to its purpose, it became the National League of Nursing Education. Miss Dock's organization admitted all graduate nurses and chose the name Associated Alumnae of the United States and Canada. Later, after a split at the border line, the American Nurses' Association emerged out of the readjustment of interests. One of its functions was to publish the *American Journal of Nursing* which became, and continues to be, a highly useful clearing house of ideas, a center for the distribution to the profession of the latest information about nursing.

The preaching of doctrine was not the only activity of these militant leaders. Wherever audiences came together to listen to discussions of the work of women, they seized the floor to urge practical and purposeful programs for improvement of the conditions under which nurses served. Such a group was the New York Federation of Women's Clubs. In 1898 Sophia Palmer told these homemakers that they must help to get legal protection for nurses in an important matter. What they wanted was the right to regulate admission to their ranks. Members of the examining board which passed on the qualifications of nurses must be chosen, not by political influence, but from among nurses themselves. And the Federation did succeed in getting them at least a part of what Sophia Palmer asked — a state law in New York which created the official post, nurse inspector of training schools.

This ferment of worker's pride produced effects in widely scattered places throughout the United States. In 1897 the University of Texas took over the John Sealy Hospital at Galveston and assumed management of its training school for nurses. Bright omen though this was considered to be, the Galveston experiment was no more a new departure than Miss Hampton's program at Johns Hopkins Hospital had been. No effort was made to put the educational work for nurses on a university level and nurses were not regarded as members of the intellectual community. They were aliens on the periphery of a university system still.

An ironic result of these small forays into the future of education was that a training program for graduate nurses came into existence, under university sponsorship, before there was any such program for beginning nurses. What may appear to be an awkward backing into progress was, in fact, an inevitable development. During the last decade of the nineteenth century training schools in hospitals multiplied many times over. There were only 35 such places in 1890; by the turn of the century there were 432. The problem of where to find superintendents to head these institutions perplexed the medical world. Someone had to undertake their special training.

Again it was Isabel Hampton who seized the initiative. In 1898 she read a paper before the Society of Superintendents calling attention to the emergency. It reached the hands of the liberal-minded dean of Teachers College, Columbia University, James E. Russell. He would open the doors to Teachers College for qualified nurses, Dean Russell said, adding, in effect, that Miss Hampton would have to do the work.

This assignment consisted in part of raising $50,000 to create the course. This stumbling block did not for long baffle women who had had wide experience in improvising projects. Driblets from here and there finally made up the entire sum. It remained only for Miss Hampton to devise the program itself. Hospital Economics was offered for the first time in 1899. The class consisted of two young women. One of them, Anna Alline, later made her own contribution to nursing history by remaining at Columbia and helping greatly to broaden its program. She served also as first inspector of nurses for the state of New York.

A prominent sharer in this new experiment was M. Adelaide Nutting. Like Miss Hampton a Canadian by birth, Miss Nutting had followed the pattern established by Florence Nightingale. She was given, at home and in private schools, the education that seemed appropriate for a child of the nineteenth century's genteel tradition. Its emphasis was on music and art. Breaking resolutely out of this mold she followed Miss Hampton's example, step by step. She was, first, Miss Hampton's pupil at Johns Hopkins; then her successor there as superintendent; later her collaborator, as one of the Committee of Three, in setting up Columbia's program; and, finally, her associate again, as head of the Department of Nursing and Health at Teachers College. In 1907 she became the first nurse to occupy a chair on a university staff. When Yale awarded her an honorary degree, many years later, the citation of distinction, written by Professor William Lyon Phelps, referred to her as "one of the most useful women in the world."

Another of these superlatively useful women who contributed abundantly, not to say lavishly, to the prestige of nursing was Lillian Wald. Her service was, quite simply, unique. A graduate of the New York Hospital School of Nursing, Miss Wald became generously obsessed with the idea of serving the abjectly poor households of New York

City's East Side. Wishing to become a better-equipped teacher, she studied medicine and then went into the tenement district to give nursing instruction to its mothers. Presently she began to identify herself completely with the people who lived in that crowded, woefully underprivileged corner of American civilization. It was not enough to go to them as philanthropic guide and counselor; she must live among them as neighbor. In Henry Street she founded her famous settlement house and became at once teacher, protector, and friend to thousands of people.

When Columbia's program of training for graduate nurses was being expanded, Lillian Wald was drawn into it. The active collaboration between settlement house and Teachers College opened up previously unimagined opportunities for training in all the complexities, all the by-paths, of nursing service.

The outlook for nursing was much improved, between 1890 and 1910, by the pioneering efforts of these most admirably useful women. But the nurse's life still demanded uncompromising abnegation of most of the comforts and graces of human experience. A young woman in training at Johns Hopkins Hospital in the 1890's worked nine hours a day (until Miss Hampton managed to get the schedule reduced to eight) and for twelve hours on night duty. A "deadening routine of repetitive tasks" (as one early graduate has described her days) was illuminated by little theoretical instruction. Anatomy and physiology were learned sketchily by examining a manikin. One hour of classroom instruction and one lecture by a doctor each week made up the progam even at the height of Miss Hampton's influence. For the rest the nurse had to be satisfied with being a docile and tireless apprentice.

Once she had been graduated from training school the nurse went into private practice. The tradition of the special-duty nurse in a hospital hardly existed. In a home she worked at wages of from $15 to $25 a week. She was on duty around the clock and was permitted time off for sleep or recreation only at the convenience of the family.

Employment agencies existed in 1900 but more often than not the nurse got her assignments in curiously casual ways. Usually she was summoned by a friendly druggist to whom an anxious father of a family had appealed for help in an emergency. If her assignments were arduous some of them had at least the advantage of semi-security.

On an obstetric case a nurse might be continued for three months, serving both as protector of the child and companion to the mother.

Her outfit consisted, as a diary of the 1900's recalls, of four voluminous, ankle-length, leg-of-mutton-sleeved uniforms; two or three reference books; and a supply of nursing appliances all crowded into a scuffed portmanteau.

This product of the average three-year training school had had experience in little beside the fundamental skills of her work. She knew, for example, no more than her individual insights could tell her about the psychological crises of family life which frequently disrupted and sometimes defeated her ministrations. She knew — and was supposed to know — little about drugs despite the fact that, as early as the turn of the century, Lillian Wald's Henry Street nurses had made a start toward carrying about with them "certain bottles and porcelain jugs" which contained soothing and pain-relieving medicaments.

The nurse traveled from home to her job in a cindery railway coach because she could afford no better. She was a laborer at heavy, exhausting duty — sometimes loved, sometimes indulgently treated at the whim of an amiable employer, but still a disciple of a harsh discipline, one who was assumed to have taken vows of poverty in the service of humanity. But what troubled her most was that she felt no inner security in the practice of her work. She simply did not know enough.

Sentimentalized as her position might be, especially by those who hoped unconsciously to exploit her desire to serve, the nurse of serious and reflective temperament felt keenly the lack of that special kind of self-respect which sustains the professional worker.

But the crusading efforts of Isabel Hampton, Adelaide Nutting, Lillian Wald, and others of their kind had not been thrown away. An atmosphere had been created in which new attitudes thrived. Out of the changes in routine which the useful women of the nineteenth century had been able to affect, an emergent profession was taking form.

For its next moment of drama the scene shifted to the Middle West where a small, determined man, member of the faculty of a good but little-known medical school, had persuaded himself that it must be his contribution to the history of education in America to prompt, urge, and stubbornly insist upon the creation of a top-level school for nurses.

1

Nestor of Nurses

✿ THE decade and a half between 1893 when Isabel Hampton Robb first called vigorously for the reform of nursing education and 1908 when Dr. Richard Olding Beard first lent an authoritative voice to the idea of establishing a university school of nursing covered a period of swift improvement for the outlook of the emergent profession. Chief catalyst of action in the movement to strengthen the whole system of instruction was Adelaide Nutting upon whom Mrs. Robb's mantle may be said to have fallen.

Miss Nutting accomplished many things: establishment of the three-year course as standard for the diploma schools; regulation of the workday for students and its limitation to eight hours; initiation of a six month's preparatory course which served as a model for many schools to follow. Her influence helped to deepen the content of science courses, to improve facilities and equipment for training, to stimulate the preparation of good textbooks, to encourage their wide use, and to make a start toward the establishment of libraries devoted to nursing literature.

But this highly significant advance for the existing schools did not satisfy her ambitions. What she wanted were major reforms: the separation of schools of nursing from hospital control and the provision of endowments or other financial support for self-regulating schools. More than all else she wanted organization of the nursing profession and recognition of its importance by universities. It was while she was engaged in campaigns, conducted through the national societies of superintendents and graduate nurses, to awaken this sense of obligation that Dr. Beard made his surprising debut as champion of the effort.

There is little obvious reason why the head of a department of physiology in a Midwestern school of medicine should have decided that he must be the person to father and foster a new experiment in education for women. Yet he did so with such effectiveness that he became, as one of his colleagues has called him, "Nestor of nurses" for the whole profession in the United States.

Dr. Beard was a tiny man with piercing black eyes, pink cheeks, a crisp style of utterance, an authoritative manner, and a goatee which, in his later years, was as opalescent-white as milk. It was his habit to stride into a classroom, read an essay on an aspect of physiology which struck his listeners as being of surprisingly bright polish, and then stride out again. He had a taste for literary reference, and the cadence of romantic theater rang through his prose.

It was brave of him to offer such lectures to his students of the early days for, by his own account, they were an amiably rugged lot with a penchant for putting dead animals on the lectern of any professor whom they did not like and for seeing to it, just on general principles, that "stiffs" were introduced regularly into faculty meetings. But "Dicky" Beard won general respect for his diminutive, yet durable, version of "patience on a monument." More than most, nurses had reason to value his qualities of protectiveness and resolution. Many references in early issues of the *American Journal of Nursing* testify to the fact that for a whole generation of nurses the face of Dr. Beard reflected the steady glow of the father image.

Born in England, Richard Beard had been brought to America at the age of thirteen. His father established the family in Chicago and, half a dozen years later, the young man entered Northwestern University Medical School. He was graduated in 1882 and moved to Minneapolis where he set himself up in the practice of medicine. Always at home on the platform, he welcomed every opportunity to discuss problems of medicine in public. After one such occasion two of the pioneer schools promptly offered him teaching jobs. Dr. Beard accepted an appointment from the Minneapolis Hospital College.

In 1888 Dr. Perry H. Millard started a movement to unify Minnesota's medical instruction in one strong institution rather than to allow effort to continue to be scattered through several weak ones. Dr.

Beard was a vigorously active member of the original group that took up the suggestion. They were successful in persuading four institutions voluntarily to surrender their charters and accept absorption into a new school sponsored by the University of Minnesota. Dr. Beard became a member of the first faculty.

This experiment was unusual in the early history of medical education in the United States. Most of what passed for training sprang out of the need of hospitals to prepare men for the immediate practical work of the wards. Minnesota's medical school began instead in the classroom, with the emphasis on theory. The "vital entity of science," as Dean Elias P. Lyon once said, must be the student's concern. It was to communicate this kind of broad interest and knowledge that the school existed, rather than merely to acquaint men with certain kinds of techniques. Because of this underlying principle, to which all members of the faculty gave willing support, the school was able to establish itself early as an able teaching unit. The Flexner report of 1910 gave it high marks, calling it one of the best institutions of its kind then in existence.

Still, for the first twenty years of its existence the medical school at Minnesota had to suffer the disadvantage of having no hospital of its own. Laboratories and space for clinical instruction were added as fast as the legislature could be persuaded to provide them. But it was not until 1905 that anyone dared to say "hospital" for fear of rousing bitter charges of extravagance. It was finally through the bounty of private citizens that a start was made toward providing an essential improvement of facilities.

Dr. Adolphus F. Elliot had been a practicing physician of Minneapolis in the city's early days. His own education had been of the rudimentary kind with which professional men had then to be content. Perhaps because he would have wished to have a better background, he took a generous interest in the university. And this interest his wife shared. After her husband's death, Mrs. Elliot created a loan fund for the use of needy students and after her own death it was found that she had left a large bequest to the university. Mrs. Elliot's will contained no stipulation as to how the money was to be used, but her executors decided that there could be no more appropriate return for this good will than to create a hospital in Dr. Elliot's name.

By present-day standards the cost of doing so was fabulous in the reverse of the more familiar sense. From the Elliot estate approximately $120,000 was realized. To this sum citizens of Minneapolis added $42,000 with which to purchase a site and the legislature promised $88,000 more for equipment. Everything went well in the planning stage and the community hoped soon to see the institution open its doors "to the needy of the State upon medical certification."

But a garrulous comedy of delay intervened between design and realization. Announcement of the Elliot bequest came in 1905 and the actual dedication of Elliot Hospital in 1911. Meanwhile history paused to listen, with what patience it could command, to the chatty discussions of protocol and procedure that so often accompany public projects.

The first delay in getting a skeleton plan decently clothed in brick resulted from a certain anxious scrupulousness on the part of the board of regents. Since the turn of the century a struggle had been going on between the president of the university and the regents, on the one side, and agencies of the state government, on the other, as to who was in actual control of the budget. The state, through its own Board of Control, had assumed the right to supervise the finances of the university as it supervised those of charitable and penal institutions. For years the university was in the humiliating position of having to petition for the right to spend its own money. Crises of Homeric proportion sprang up over such issues as the expenditure of fifteen cents for paraffin needed by a teacher of engineering for purposes of demonstration in one of his classes.

The situation became steadily worse until President Cyrus Northrop, a man of great personal power and prestige, went before the legislature, like a Priam, to ransom the body of the budget from the statehouse. Armed with his own unassailable integrity he carried the limp, tormented, and exhausted form home to the campus.

Yet, although the board of regents was "authorized by statute to receive gifts to the university," its members hesitated in the matter of the Elliot bequest to act without the special permission of the state. For this they had to wait until the 1907 session. And while they waited the old improvising practices in medical instruction went on.

There were other frustrating delays. One of these was caused, as President Northrop reported with what was for him an almost unknown note of asperity, by an unaccountable delay in designing a new area of the campus and "locating the buildings upon it."

Despite these annoyances the vision of the non-existent hospital stood clear in the minds of long-range planners. One of these, of course, was Dr. Beard. He was thinking of the school for nurses that the university must have to go with its new hospital.

He had been a fluent theorist on the subject of education for many years. And in all his discussions he included the right of the nurse to a good education, along with the right of the teacher and that of the physician. The state university which, as he said, is "the college of the people" must train all those whose task it is to conserve "human life, human development and human health." Through "its highest educational agencies" it must provide suitable preparation.

The announcement that the University of Minnesota had decided to sponsor the first program for the education of the nurse on the collegiate level was made by Dr. Beard before a joint meeting of the Society of Superintendents of Training Schools for Nurses and the Associated Alumnae of the United States and Canada. The session was held in Minneapolis and among its attendants was Mrs. Robb. Both she and Dr. Beard remembered the occasion as the history-making event that it actually was. For Mrs. Robb it was something more besides. As she told Dr. Beard "the dream of her life" was about to be fulfilled. Quite unapologetically she wept "tears that came from a deep gratitude."

Down the years, later commentators have taken the same view. As one historian, Deborah MacLurg Jensen, has said, the establishment of the first university school of nursing was "a step of the greatest consequence for nursing education. It changed the status of the fledgling nurse from that of a 'pupil nurse' to that of a student. The final step in the creation of the nursing *profession* had been taken."

The first anticipatory action toward the conduct of a non-existent school, attached by the link of imagination to a hospital that had still to be built, was to appoint a superintendent of nurses. A graduate nurse, Bertha Erdmann, was chosen and the selection was a good one. Miss Erdmann had close associations with the academic world through a brother, Dr. Charles A. Erdmann, who was long a valuable member of the medical faculty. She understood the temper of the university well; when the Advisory Committee suggested that she might like to do graduate work before taking up her post she went obediently to Columbia.

There she talked with the enthusiasm which had become standard equipment for men and women of the Minnesota project about the new experiment in nursing education which was to admit young women who could meet the entrance requirements of the university. Among those to whom she talked was a fellow student, Miss Louise Powell, who — as it turned out — was to become her successor in conducting that same experiment.

On the campus Dr. Beard was stirring about with the energy needed to put a roof over a vision and enclose it within four walls. As he was later to write: "We did not despise the day of small things." The small things that had to be accepted in place of the hospital promised for the future were the frame buildings at 200 and 304 State Street and at 303 Washington Avenue — old dwellings, they were hastily converted into hospital units. One had been used as the chapter house of Phi Kappa Psi until the fraternity had achieved greater grandeur.

Washington Avenue is one of the thoroughfares of interurban traffic between Minneapolis and St. Paul which cuts off slices of the campus, here and there. Its strenuous busyness quite irremediably destroys any effect of academic seclusion, yet it symbolizes, not at all unwelcomely, the close link of the university to the community. Today, the "new campus," and the towering buildings of the medical center line it. But in 1909 a village atmosphere prevailed and it would have been difficult for the most dedicated visionary of the period to foresee the present development.

The official date of the opening of the School for Nurses, as it was originally called, is March 1, 1909. It began actually to function a few days later. Its staff consisted of "one trained nurse and two assistants." Members of the faculty of the medical school were its teachers except for instruction in "nursing arts" which Miss Erdmann taught in the midst of a flurry of administrative duties. Dr. Beard was directly "in charge of arrangements."

The hospital, to which everyone hopefully referred as "temporary," was housed in the most adaptable of the old houses. Wards were set up in made-over livingrooms and bedrooms. There were accommodations for twenty-five patients. The operating room was, as a later reporter confessed, "so crude that it would be hard to believe good nursing could be done in it." The staircase was narrow and precipitous. A stretcher could not be managed on it and sturdy internes from the

Minnesota farms had to carry patients in their arms from the operating room back to their beds. The rest of the facilities consisted of a delivery room, a room for two internes, and a kitchen in which food for patients could be heated. (Meals were prepared in a house several blocks away.) The street door opened into a front hall where, within easy access of all the drafts from Washington Avenue and all its noises as well, stood the desks of the superintendent of nurses and that of the secretary of the hospital superintendent. This was the beginning and the end of that first shadowing forth of a university hospital.

The three-year program which Miss Erdmann inaugurated was similar to that designed by Professor Nutting and adopted by the more advanced schools of the time. But there were differences which made it unique. First, it had the enormous advantage of association with the able teaching unit of the medical school. Second, despite its poverty, it was required to be highly selective in admission of students. These had to be not only of superior educability but of greater stability in temperament as well. No candidate was admitted unless she were interested in achieving something more than a means of livelihood. The university was seeking — and got — women who wanted careers in nursing. Finally, the whole project was wrapped up in the atmosphere of prestige that attaches to a university experiment. For all its hazards and inconveniences this had become an occupation and a way of life of which a young woman could be proud.

Miss Erdmann's excellent reports show that she had every intention of preserving all these advantages. She was resolute in turning away those who did not "belong."

Unfortunately, she was able to stay at her job only a year. Personal tragedy took her to a hospital as a patient where, far too young, she died of tuberculosis.

And presently Louise Powell stood in her place.

Miss Powell was just under forty years old when she came to Minnesota in July, 1910, and she had a good background of preparation and experience. Born in Staunton, Virginia, a small community which fifteen years earlier had produced Woodrow Wilson, Louise Powell had attended a local school and then, like so many of her distinguished predecessors in the nursing field — Florence Nightingale, Isabel Hampton, Adelaide Nutting — had begun her career as a teacher of grade-school children. Then, in her late twenties, in response to the instinctual impulse toward social service which had led the others into nursing, she began all over. She was graduated from St. Luke's Hospital at Richmond, Virginia, in 1899 and was for five subsequent years its superintendent of nurses. Later she was the infirmary nurse at Baldwin School, Bryn Mawr, until she decided to take the graduate course at Columbia. All her life Miss Powell worked conscientiously at improving her qualifications as educator. For her it was the perfect holiday to take postgraduate work at the Hospital for Sick Children at Mt. Wilson, Maryland, at the Municipal Hospital for Contagious Diseases at Philadelphia, or even on the less interestingly plague-ridden campuses of the University of Virginia, Columbia, and Smith College.

All her life, too, Miss Powell spoke with the soft accent of her birthplace and with the overtone of humor. A sister, whose name, Lucy Lee, testified to a close connection with the famous Lee family of which both Powells were very proud, also came to Minnesota, to serve the Minneapolis Public Library.

These ladies delighted in each other's society and in the fact that each was, in her way, dedicated to the work of education. But, as an associate of their early days in Minneapolis has recalled, they would occasionally become depressed by their lack of worldly success. Brooding on the inevitable end that awaited their hopes they would sit down together and write their wills. But they had never been at this sad business long when other nurses would hear peals of laughter emanating from Miss Louise's room. Then her words would come clear through the laughter: "But, sistah, this is absurd. We have *nothing* to leave to *anybody*."

Miss Powell had received her Minnesota appointment at the suggestion of her teacher, Adelaide Nutting. Miss Nutting had moved toward her administrative post in the footsteps of Isabel Hampton. So, in a kind of apostolic succession, the determination to improve the outlook for nursing was passed along and transported to Minnesota as though it were part of the paraphernalia in Miss Powell's portmanteau.

Yet when she began her assignment she must have felt that the atmosphere, blended of future hope and present penury, would keep her vibrating dizzily between expectation and despair. As she herself later reported, conditions in the nurses' home were dismally primitive. She remembered it — though not with love — "for its entire lack of privacy and comfort, for the radiators that sounded like a bombardment and the smell of the laundry which met you" — again, not like a friend — "as you entered the front door."

Miss Powell, having survived all these attacks on the sensibilities, recalled, with the poet's tranquillity chiefly, how hopeful she and her students were. As they broke their way through block after block of snowdrifts, still unshoveled at the early hour when they rose to go to breakfast in a distant house, their spirits seldom wavered, even though Minnesota's subzero weather must often have made the pilgrimage seem like martyrdom.

"However, we could see the walls of the hospital building rising over on the river," Miss Powell concluded her remembrance, "and we could laugh at our inconveniences and think that they were temporary and soon there would be an elevator so that patients would not have to be carried to and from the operating room, up and down stairs, and that food and laundry could be easily transported from floor to floor."

2

Adventure in Education

ꙮ THE attempt to conduct an experiment in education is often beset at the start by baffling difficulties which tend to defeat its essential
purpose. An impulse reveals itself, here or there, to allow a new idea
to be contaminated by concession. There are pressing and plausible
influences which would urge a turning away from the untried, back
toward practices and procedures which no one would call ideal but
which have the advantage of familiarity.

Following the debut of the nursing school at Minnesota, Miss Powell
and her advisers faced many such difficulties. As they might have said,
the first eight years were the hardest.

What sustained Miss Powell's determination to follow the instruction of her teacher, Professor Nutting, was the fact that she had the
support of two men who valued her principles and were always ready
to help her fight for them. Dr. Beard was constantly at her side — and
on her side — in any contest over standards. Equally important to her
was the steady and reliable cooperation of Dr. Louis Baldwin who had
been appointed by the board of regents to be superintendent of Elliot
Hospital a year before the building actually existed.

Dr. Baldwin was an organizer of unusual capability. Not only did
he design and re-design the complex pattern of facilities at the university, as these developed rapidly during the later years of his administration ; he also went on part-time loan, in another period, to establish a plan for the management of the Charles T. Miller Hospital in
St. Paul. He was, in fact, collaborator on two systems of patient care

and student instruction which were of the greatest importance to the community.

In a retrospective glance at her Minnesota years Miss Powell once paid grateful tribute to the "splendid team work" during the early years of "discomforts and inconveniences" when she and Dr. Baldwin "worked together in perfect harmony." The superintendent of the hospital had, she said, "as fair a mind as I ever knew." And she added:

"Once convinced that a demand was reasonable he put all his energy to work to get it granted. He had, to an unusual degree, the ability to delegate authority to those in charge of departments and would leave them to work out problems according to their own ideas — ready always to cooperate."

The problems with which Miss Powell, Dr. Beard, and Dr. Baldwin struggled were of several kinds. There was, first, that of attracting the kind of "quality student" whom a university school of nursing could accept; second, that of establishing a curriculum and broadening facilities of instruction; third, that of making do with inadequate housing for nurses; fourth, that of the formidable load of their own responsibilities; and, fifth, that of countering objections to the program which came, sometimes, even from members of the medical staff.

Dr. Beard, who found the atmosphere of the forum highly congenial, was Miss Powell's spokesman in many a campaign to keep standards of admission high. Like Professor Nutting, he wanted to see schools of nursing removed from the rigid and arbitrary control of hospitals. In the days before 1893, when nurses themselves had begun to create a demand for a higher level of training, there had been many wretched "diploma factories." Remembering them, Dr. Beard called for a break with the past when instruction had served often to "emphasize the unfitness of the originally unfit." The superintendent of a hospital in New York City, he observed on one occasion, had admitted that, in a class of sixty probationers, thirty had had poor qualifications for entrance by the school's own standards, yet they had been accepted simply because the institution "had to have them." It would be possible to tempt women back into the profession only if they were assured that they would be given a genuine education, one that would train them "thoroughly and broadly to fill the important place they should occupy in the community."

It followed inevitably that there must be careful selection of students, for only able ones could profit by the kind of program Dr. Beard wanted to see established. It is interesting to notice that he made the approach to the problem which would suggest itself only to a staunch feminist. In a day when the idea of "votes for women" was still regarded as a merely laughable aberration on the part of certain over-zealous cranks, Dr. Beard dared to suggest that "among enlightened people" attitudes even toward the work of the housewife were being fundamentally revised. "Woman," he said, "is coming to choose marriage not, as in the past, because there is nothing else for her to do, but as her highest choice." To be free to make such a choice she must have a vocation of her own. If "the practice of nursing is to become such a vocation," Dr. Beard insisted, it must "be elevated by a course of preparation" that would give the able woman a secure command of her responsibilities.

To the job of finding the superior student Miss Powell lent all her powers of concentrated effort. She was a small woman but her sense of responsibility was enormous and she found the energy to match the high peak of her resolution. For days on end she would sit in the drafty hall consulting with candidates, weighing, with them, their qualifications, their interest, and their adaptability.

In the day of the catch-as-catch-can system when training schools took applicants because they "had to have them," it had been a simple matter to gain admission. A young woman presented herself to a superintendent of nurses and if she looked healthy she was told to return next day with a supply of "plain wash dresses and white aprons." At seven thirty in the morning she reported to a head nurse who showed her how to make a bed, how to "dust" by wiping all the objects in the ward with water that smelled of carbolic acid, and how in the course of nine hours of heavy labor to discover in her own exhausted, aching body muscles and ligaments the existence of which she had never before suspected. And this was the whole of the introductory process. She was now a student nurse.

Very different were the procedures of Miss Powell and Dr. Beard, who sat on the entrance committee.

First, a young woman who hoped to become a student nurse at Minnesota had to send her high school credentials to the registrar's office. If these were acceptable her name was added to a list of candidates sent to the superintendent's desk. Each of these was notified of the day and hour when she must appear before the entrance committee on the campus. It was a searching investigation of her past, present, and future that she met on that first day in the university world.

Before she could even be considered as an applicant for admission she must undergo a physical examination. If any serious defect seemed to appear she was asked to report to the hospital for a more thorough investigation. Only when she had passed these tests could she sit down with the entrance committee and let them explore her individual qualities. The members wanted what a modern counselor would call "a personality profile of the subject."

The purpose of all this was not to baffle or humiliate ambition but rather to try to insure success. The University of Minnesota was committed firmly and forever to the policy of taking all suitable material. But it was beginning already to make the discriminating effort at proper placement for which the psychological testing bureau was later to become famous.

Even after a student was accepted her performance was carefully watched. At various phases the record of each student was reviewed by the superintendent. More was taken into account than simply classroom grades. It was still necessary to weed out those who had come to the school simply to find a shortcut to livelihood and who took little interest in the theoretical aspects of instruction. Harder to identify were those whose ability to learn was sufficient but whose sensibilities were at war, in this work, with ambition. It was necessary also to discourage those whose sense of vocation had in it too much ecstasy and too little of inclination toward science. Over the years Miss Powell earned the reputation of being as considerate as she was firm. The most demure and feminine of judges ever to earn the description Rhadamantine, she forced herself to send away many a girl to another occupation.

In building up the curriculum of the school the members of the advisory committee had taken, as foundation, the three-year program suggested by the pioneers of nursing education, particularly those at Teachers College, Columbia. But to these they added important extensions of their own, drawing on the resources of the university system to broaden instruction and enlarge opportunity. They even reached beyond the campus to find fields of study that opened up a larger outlook for the nurse.

The young matriculant took first the "preparatory course," that bridge between the experiences of high school and those of professional experience the strategic importance of which Professor Nutting had been the first to see. This offered her a general view of her field and introducd her to some of the scientific subjects with which her later courses were to be concerned. The second semester of her first year was spent studying anatomy, physiology, chemistry, materia medica, and hospital economics. In the earliest period the student was treated, during the probationary course, like a freshman in any other college: she paid tuition and did no hospital duty. But before the end of Miss Powell's regime conditions and practices had changed. Even in her first year, the student was assigned to duty and received instruction in the men's and women's surgical wards of the hospital.

During the other two years of training, the student nurse's basic subjects were:

SECOND YEAR

Surgical nursing .... 19 hours
Bandaging .... 6 hours
Gynecology .... 5 hours
Obstetrics .... 7 hours
Physiologic chemistry .... 3 hours

THIRD YEAR

Dietetics .... 24 hours
Practical nursing................... 13 hours
Massage .... 24 hours
Nervous and mental................. 5 hours
Eye, ear, nose, and throat............ 4 hours
Applied dietetics................... 3 hours

Lectures in clinical subjects were given by members of the medical faculty. Teachers of practice classes were the graduate nurses who headed the wards of the hospital. Though these women were not, as their counterparts are today, highly trained in teaching methods, Miss Powell felt that because of their wide experience they had "much to give the young students."

Besides being a conscientious pioneer educator, Miss Powell was herself a tireless student. It was her delight as well as her task to provide stimulation for her students and, in doing so, she helped to open up new areas of study. Remembering her own work with sick children, she encouraged the development of a new course called Invalid Occupation, intended "to teach nurses the importance of keeping the convalescent patient pleasantly entertained." Step by step she explored the advantages of the school's position within a large university system and added to the curriculum such experiences as that of service in the dental clinic where students "learned the value of oral hygiene to general health." In 1916 she persuaded a member of the sociology department to give an introductory course "especially designed for nurses." These were modest, yet significant, experiments representing a consistent movement toward today's idea of training the nurse for "total care" of the patient.

Another contribution toward the same goal was made when the advisory committee of the school voted, in 1917, to enter into an affiliation with Glen Lake Tuberculosis Sanatorium. It had become Miss Powell's conviction that the services of Elliot Hospital were too limited to awaken a full understanding of the psychology of the patient. Many weeks of routine practice in medical and surgical departments were, she thought, likely to have a deadening effect. To be exposed to new ideas, new procedures, and new experiments was what students needed to make their work meaningful.

At that moment, in an institution just a few miles away from the campus, a distinguished man was beginning to put new techniques and, what was more important, new attitudes, at the service of the tuberculosis patient. Dr. Ernest Sidney Mariette was a pioneer of method in the physical treatment of the disease itself. He was acutely aware also of the truth, made clear by Thomas Mann in *The Magic Mountain*, that tuberculosis imposes on its victims a special way of life. Because, in his opinion, nurses were as important as doctors themselves to the work of encouraging helpful attitudes, not only to patients but to the members of their families, he had long been an advocate of better education for women. The significance of Dr. Mariette's innovations was so widely recognized that Glen Lake Sanatorium was the first institution of its kind in the United States to be accredited by the American Medical Association.

The school established a two-month period of service, under Dr. Mariette's instruction and guidance. Students were assigned to it as a regular part of the training course.

Allied to Miss Powell's desire to offer students as liberal an experience as possible was her determination to see that all courses were taught thoroughly. Standards, she told the advisory committee, were bound to deteriorate under a system in which an instructor in nursing arts must split herself up a dozen ways. The practice of nursing, she said, "can be taught only by a nurse who has time to teach all procedures in the classroom and then follow up the nurses in the wards to see that they are doing the work as they have been taught."

Early in the teens of the century, when she began to feel solid ground under her feet, Miss Powell began to urge the appointment of an assistant teacher. But she wanted "the proper person," one who must be paid — let the gentlemen resign themselves to this extravagance as best they could! — "not less than $75 a month."

The proper person was found at last. Elizabeth Pierce came to Minnesota from Teachers College, Columbia. She had received her early training at the Jewish Hospital Training School in Cincinnati and was then at the beginning of a career which was to make her conspicuous in the field of pediatric nursing. With her she brought a large supply of the invisible but indispensable equipment of the nurse: enthusiasm, sympathy, and high spirit. She made, as Miss Powell's reports testify, an important contribution to "the friendly atmosphere that was prevalent in the School and the Hospital in those early years."

As a sort of alter ego to the indestructibly cheerful superintendent herself Miss Pierce lent eyes, ears, and understanding to the job of keeping students pleased with their work. And this was important, Miss Powell insisted; for the future of nursing depended on its ability to attract and hold a stable and mature type of student.

Miss Pierce was herself the sort of superior product whose services other institutions were bound to covet. In a first tour of duty she stayed at Minnesota only a year. (She was later to return in a time of great emergency.) But again Miss Powell was able to find an appropriate successor. Marion L. Vannier came with the idea of staying six months while Miss Powell went on one of her periodic leaves to engage in study; she remained for a decade and a half, first as assistant superintendent, later as Miss Powell's successor.

"A figure of Dresden china elegance and poise," as she has been called by an associate, Miss Vannier had vigor to match her social grace and decisiveness to balance suavity. "The very great lady with the aquiline nose" was another description offered, in rueful admiration, by a doctor who had been politely worsted in an argument over school policy. For Miss Vannier, too, could be firm when she felt that matters of educational principle were at stake.

Another touchingly modest effort to improve facilities resulted in the establishment of a library of nursing literature. Reference works and magazines were "put at the disposal of nurses in a corner of the medical library." To it men of the medical faculty made donations and Dr. James T. Gerould — then in the process of building up the university's now distinguished library — showed, as Miss Powell reported, "unfailing willingness" to buy such books as she recommended.

In the first years of its existence the school followed the difficult course of adventure. But those who charted the course did not lose faith in the possibility of attaining their objective. Realization of Dr. Beard's own ideal of what a university school of nursing should be was still to come. But if progress was slow and uncertain, at least the navigators were determined not to turn back.

But the problem of housing continued to be acute. Despite their readiness to improvise in many ways, the women of the school found it by no means easy to accept the humble way of life they must live in private. To work hard, under difficulties, for the ultimate good of the school was a stimulating experience. But to go at the end of the exhausting day's work to a wayward little extension of Grub Street — this was a trial of the nerves that became steadily more exacerbating.

When the school first opened nurses were told that their housing arrangements were "temporary." But the years, "like black oxen," plodded doggedly on and on without any changes being made. The nursing population was still scattered through many houses, all equally unpleasant.

The full capacity of the homes on Delaware and Church Streets was reached and, as classes increased in numbers, the superintendent never knew, from semester to semester, where students would lay their heads. Thirty-two nurses lived at one moment in what had been a modest family residence; ten of them slept in five tiny rooms, eleven feet square, each with one window, no door transom, and one closet. Sixteen more young women lived in quarters made over from diningroom and kitchen and they had no closet space at all. In a grotesque tenement parade nurses moved back and forth daily through each other's rooms to reach bathroom and storage areas. The building was lighted by gas and even this concession to modern luxury was made without lavish generosity.

There was only one burner to a room. The "cottages on Church Street" sounded as though they might have been left over from some idyll of country life, but they were distinctly nothing of the sort. The heating, Miss Powell confided to Dr. Beard in a report marked throughout by heroic understatement, was not satisfactory in cold weather because "the janitor finds it hard to regulate in addition to his other work." The furnaces were not fired "early enough to make the house comfortable at 5:45" at which hour the nurses were called. The hot water supply was "irregular and hard to manage."

Patiently, Miss Powell recorded the opinion that these conditions were "unsanitary and unhygienic in the extreme." The lack of privacy alone was "nerve wearing;" the entire way of life was "absolutely unfit for women subjected to the nervous strain of nursing for 56 hours a week."

It was clear to Miss Powell that this was far too heavy a schedule and she took a brisk little shortcut toward progress. In instances where quick action was required she could show a firm unobtrusiveness that baffled resistance. This was such an occasion. Miss Powell simply reduced the workweek to 48 hours without, as she confessed much later, "bothering to consult anyone."

In many other ways Miss Powell helped to alleviate the Spartan discipline of the early days. In the wards she could be an exacting taskmistress and students were not sorry that she wore at her waist a watch the very loud ticking of which warned them of her approach. But in the nurses' home she never neglected what she considered to be her duties as foster mother to a large brood. Not only did she encourage her students to find amusement; she added to her heavy schedule of responsibilities by undertaking to provide it. Early graduates of the school value the image of Miss Powell as a winsome bride in a mock wedding. By such adroit and timely surrenders of dignity she helped to keep the atmosphere of the school intimate and familial. This solidarity of temper, established at the start, has not been lost since. Its pervasive influence in the early years was of genuine importance in helping a small school to grow.

An event of that period attractively dramatized the school's *esprit de corps.* A new group of students was greeted by an impromptu fair. There was dancing in Essex Street, and two internes made a contribution to the robust temper of such a traditional celebration by putting on a wrestling match. Visitors arrived from all corners of the campus, curious to see what the sport was about. Such efforts were not without significance to the educational program for they tended to make the young nurse feel that she was really a student in the university, not a stranger living on the periphery of its social life.

A Cratchit-like vein of resolute cheerfulness ran through all these efforts to create a pleasant atmosphere. Successes were as modest as the response to them was enthusiastic. Once Miss Powell was able to persuade the sister of a graduate to give a piano to the nurses' home. She made a personal appeal to friends for contributions to "a good fiction library." Acting consciously on the theory that "social gatherings" are "most important in the lives of women whose daily program is as strenuous and often as depressing as is that of the nurse," she urged the establishment of "a small fund with which to provide occasional entertainment." With a kind of soft persistence she pursued her plans up every promising bypath. One of her reports suggests: "We can give a dance in Shevlin Hall for about $12 and I feel that this should be done about three times a year with an outdoor party in summer."

With this far from riotous schedule of pleasures Miss Powell was prepared to make do. But the meagerness of the general living conditions still weighed heavily on her conscience. The university, she said bluntly, was being "unfair to nurses who are giving 7400 hours of service to the hospital in addition to an outlay of $150 [tuition fees]." In return students were supposed to get an education and proper housing. One report concluded: "We are most certainly not living up to our contract."

Yet there the matter rested for many years to come.

The fourth problem of the early years was Miss Powell's very own. It sprang from the obligation not merely to double in brass, but to triple, quadruple, and then still multiply her responsibilities. An adaptable pioneer in an experiment that was as poor as it was ambitious, she had to serve simultaneously as administrator, teacher, housekeeper, dietitian, quiz-master, and counselor. She planned meals for patients and nursing staff, did her own marketing by telephone and learned, as she went along, the mystique of northern cookery in contrast to her own southern style. She taught courses in the practice of nursing, at first quite without equipment. She attended the lectures of the doctors in order to be able to conduct examinations in all the subjects of the course. At every hour of the day Miss Powell had to be ready to split the difference between administrator and teacher.

But split it she did. Though there was nothing in the least flamboyant about her style of expression, she had a distinct sense of drama; one of her reports offers an exhausting account of how she attempted to be all things to all students. A single day's schedule required her to meet the preparatory class from eleven until noon, the probationers from one o'clock to three, juniors from four to five, and seniors from five to six. From these efforts to maintain something like academic discipline in the study of nursing problems she was frequently called to the telephone to deal with crises in the hospital, with the problems of administration, or simply the details that fell on the shoulders of the foster mother of a large household.

Year after year the problems remained. But so did the school, and from the standpoint of Miss Powell and her advisers, survival was a kind of triumph.

The problems of partnership with the medical school ran concurrently with all the others through the first eight years. Chief of these was the old familiar one of finding nurses to fill posts in the hospital.

An immediate effect of the decision to keep standards of admission high was to keep enrollment low. In the fall of 1910 only four women were accepted for the preparatory course and, in February, 1911, when a new semester was about to begin there were no applicants at all. Doctors, looking forward to the opening of Elliot Hospital in the fall of the same year, were understandably worried about how its 120 beds were to be served. The committee of the school met in great perturbation to look for a solution.

As Miss Powell had feared they would do, the men of the committee, each of whom headed one of the services of the hospital, agreed that, in order to meet this emergency, standards of admission must be lowered. Any applicant, the doctors urged, should be accepted who could meet the requirements of other training schools even though she could not meet those of the university. Then, later, when it was convenient, standards could be raised once more.

This would have been to betray the principle on which the school had been established in the first place. What was worse, it would have been to betray the faith of students who had come to the university in the confidence that they were being enrolled for a superior kind of education. What if there were only four of them? Miss Powell demanded briskly; they represented the future which the experiment was supposed to champion. Indeed, to have accepted this compromise would have been to go back to the beginning with nothing gained at all.

Against the immediate threat to the school's integrity and against possible demands for concession that might be made tomorrow and the day after, the triumvirate of Beard, Baldwin, and Powell took a firm stand. Instead, they suggested that the school should receive a group of nurses from St. Mary's Hospital, at Rochester, Minnesota, who were willing to come for special work in medical nursing. Unlike the university's own students these were to be paid what they would have received in their own hospital. To this the administrative committee of the school agreed, at last, though with pained reluctance.

So, in the first of the school's battles of theory versus practical advantage, theory won a total victory. The men of the medical school must have retired in some confusion, for almost immediately they capitulated without starting any more campaigns and decided to allow the school to run its own affairs. In the noncommittal tone which official records often adopt, for fear, perhaps, of opening old wounds, history states that the advisory committee of the school was "subsequently reorganized." No longer were there many representatives of the medical school among its members. In large matters of administrative planning, as well as in details of daily management, control was in the hands of the triumvirate.

Another conflict of interest arose, however, over the use of facilities. Though Miss Powell was "considered to be an instructor of the university," as one of her brisk reports sets forth the problem, she was given no classroom to call her own. She shared the hospital lecture room with the medical faculty and, though she made a schedule at the beginning of each year which showed the hours when she would need a room, she could never be quite sure of its availability. A busy doctor, who had missed a class and wished to make it up at exactly Miss Powell's hour, would pre-empt it. Her activities "interfered with those of the medical staff who wished to use the room for clinical teaching and she with them" so that there was "constant conflict."

But, again, it was not the personal inconvenience that mattered. The real problem was that teaching effectiveness was being destroyed. Stung for once to strong expression, the superintendent wrote:

When I teach practical nursing, fully an hour must be spent in gathering from the hospital the things needed. A bed must be rolled in; then everything must be removed at the end of the class hour. There is no place for the nurses to practice except in the wards on the patient, the very thing that we claim not to do. I have realized that we are a young institution that cannot expect to get everything at once; but I feel that the time has come to protest against any further delay in providing a decent comfortable home for the School of Nurses with adequate teaching equipment such as is given to other university departments. If we cannot do this we had better close our school and cease claiming that our School for Nurses is a university department.

But the challenge was a purely oratorical one, intended to relieve a feeling of pressure. Miss Powell went on conscientiously fighting the battle of the day of small things. As she undertook to correct old injustices and achieve unity of procedure in the daily work of the nurse there were often groans of protest at innovation. Particularly unwelcome to the doctors was the decision that there must be no more lectures at night. It had seemed to the medical staff to be the inalienable right of its members to choose their own hours for meeting classes of student nurses. Afternoon sessions interfered with office hours (and possibly with golf).

"However," says one of Miss Powell's crisp reports, "the change was made and until the next time, when something different from what they had always done, was proposed, everybody was happy."

At the end of the first eight years of its operation the outlook for the school had improved greatly. The opening of Elliot Hospital, in September, 1911, had written finis to the pioneer phase of nursing history at Minnesota. No longer did students have to sterilize their instruments by dropping them into an enamel basin filled with burning alcohol. No longer did they draw sterile water from a spigot attached to a bulky boiler in the operating room. No longer did they have to stand in fear and trembling while internes with more strength than finesse carried patients up and down stairs on their backs. Facilities were good and they continued steadily to be expanded thanks to the legislature's pride in the medical school. By 1913 Elliot Hospital had reached a capacity of 192 beds.

The problem of enrollment had been partially solved. This was not a new one in University of Minnesota history. For years it had maintained a College of Agriculture without being able to attract more than one or two students at a time out of the wheatfields into the classroom. (Often there were none at all.) For a period of fifteen years after its creation on paper, the College of Engineering was able to graduate a dismaying average of one student a year from its course though this was constantly expanded in a spirit of hopeful challenge to indifference. American democracy, despite its theoretical dedication to the values of education, had often betrayed a curious dubiety about entrusting its sons and daughters to professors who taught the work of the professions "by the book."

In comparison, the nursing school had been fortunate. In February, 1911, there were seven applicants for admission, of whom five were accepted. In September of that year, the two beginning classes, together with a group of graduate nurses entered for refresher courses, brought enrollment to fifteen. To step up numbers a little more still the committee decided to admit to the preparatory course nurses from other training schools which had no such instruction to offer. With these "affiliating students" added, the population of the school was thirty-two in the year 1914–15. In the following fall it passed the half-hundred mark.

"When we consider our high entrance requirements," Miss Powell wrote in her 1916 report, "I think we may feel encouraged."

The source from which the school was to receive its next powerful impulse toward maturity must have startled the members of the committee as they sat earnestly intent on the problems of survival. On April 16, 1917, the Congress of the United States declared war on the imperial German government. Straightway there began one of those forcing processes that allow to nations, institutions, and men no alternative but to accept new and staggering responsibilities. In its small corner of a world at war the nursing school at the University of Minnesota stood ready to take up its share of an enormous obligation.

3

Days of Disaster, Years of Growth

✿ DURING April of that year teachers found it difficult to keep to their subjects, and many a session of a course in botany, mathematics or harmony would have sounded to a casual visitor like one in contemporary European history. In and out of the classroom discussion kept looping back to the German people's fear of encirclement, to the trade war between Germany and England and to "unrestricted submarine warfare." Young men ignored the invitation of the first spring day to take the nearest attractive girl "river-banking" and wandered off in earnest knots of abstraction, talking about enlistment. Presently the campuses were decimated.

There was the greatest confusion among guardians of the classic subjects about what came next. (How could you justify a preoccupation with Beowulf in the midst of times that tried men's souls so urgently?) There was less dismay among nurses than in many another group, faced with the new responsibilities of war. The word of emergency was not new to the nurse. Her duty in this newest and greatest emergency was clear. She must continue, at quickened speed, the work that she had been prepared or was preparing to do.

By mid-August, 1917, a subcommittee of the Council of National Defense was actively at work, under the chairmanship of Adelaide Nutting, creating a pattern for the emergency training of nurses "in this great crisis." Miss Nutting's report to the superintendents of the country pointed out that the "needs of our army abroad" would probably claim, within a year, all of the twelve thousand well qualified trained nurses then enrolled for call by the Red Cross. The loss of service to the civilian community could be endured by sacrifice, adjustment, and improvisation. But the war situation served to make evident a serious dearth of workers in this field. Its leaders had been aware for a long time that the rapid development of the modern hospital and of public health work in the United States had not been supported by the needed increase in the supply of nurses — ones, especially, with a high degree of training who could "direct the nursing departments of our several thousand hospitals, organize and conduct the complicated system of training in our 1500 training schools for nurses, guide the great new field of public health in which nurses are playing so vital a part."

Miss Nutting's report went on:

Since training schools are our one source of supply for every form of real nursing work . . . [we are] suddenly brought face to face with the seriousness of the situation and the urgent necessity of prompt action. We must bring into our schools a very large number of pupils and bring them now. This is imperative . . . If we can add two or three thousand good recruits to our body of pupil-nurses during the coming year we shall go far toward settling the problem of nursing in so far as the war is concerned and we shall also be making a solid contribution toward the enlargement of the regular nursing forces of the country which will still be needed if the war should end tomorrow.

It is significant of the temper of the nursing profession that though it was actively concerned about the immediate emergency, it managed to keep long-range objectives clear. The future of the work itself was the consideration of continuing importance. The impetus of present need must be used to give the movement toward full professional status another spurt forward.

The committee on nursing appointed by the Council of National Defense already had launched a campaign to recruit, for training, young women who were recent graduates of college. Appeals had gone out to deans and their students, to public and private institutions, to superintendents of training schools — many more than 100,000 letters in all — urging an immediate response to this patriotic summons.

And the response came. The School for Nurses at Minnesota felt its effect in a twenty-five per cent increase in enrollment. This did not make the figure dazzlingly high, of course — there were sixty-nine students during the academic year 1917–18 — but even this number was sufficiently overwhelming. For the influx of matriculants came just at the moment when a symbolic swinging door facilitated the departure of the hospital staff into war service. Miss Powell, just back from a six-month leave, found the medical community at the university in the process of completing its organization of a unit to go overseas.

The university base hospital was, in fact, just five days older than the war itself. The period of its pre-history had begun a year before. In October, 1916, the surgeon general of the United States, William C. Gorgas, had anticipated the probability of America's being drawn into the struggle and had asked Dr. Will Mayo to make a start toward medical preparedness. Dr. Mayo had suggested that the University of Minnesota, as a public institution, would be the proper place at which to organize a hospital unit. With characteristic generosity, he offered to find fifty per cent of the professional personnel in the Mayo Clinic and to contribute fifty per cent of the necessary financial support.

Dr. Arthur A. Law of the university faculty assumed direct responsibility for the creation of the University Base Hospital, Unit 26. On April 1, the day before President Wilson made his eloquent speech urging Congress to declare that a state of war existed, Washington asked that the base hospital be put immediately into working order. With the speed that democracy can show when its pugnacity is aroused by challenge these steps followed:

By April 18, citizens of Minneapolis had raised $15,000 to match the sum donated by the Mayos: the Red Cross had given $10,000 worth of surgical supplies; and the unit had a solid foundation under it.

By July 1, officers, enlisted men, and nurses had been recruited to full strength and Dr. Baldwin, as volunteer purchasing agent, had assembled all necessary equipment.

By July 10, Dr. Law (recently commissioned major) was able to notify Washington that the Base Hospital, Unit 26, was ready for active duty.

Inevitably the old army game of "hurry up and wait" had thereafter to take its tedious course. It was not until December 13 that the unit received orders actually to mobilize for transfer to Fort McPherson and it was not until June 3, 1918, that the organization boarded the *Baltic* at New York, to sail for England. They had been joined there by the nurses, who sailed with the same convoy.

In its final form the unit consisted of the men from Minnesota with another group from Texas attached to bring the personnel to a number sufficient to care for a 1,000-bed hospital. The nurse corps was composed of sixty-five women from Minnesota, together with twenty nurses from the Texas unit and fifteen more who were added in New York.

Among these sixty-five citizens of Minnesota in the nurse corps, thirteen were from the School for Nurses at the university. During the year of preparation between April, 1917, and April, 1918, every head nurse in the school who was physically fit had been accepted to go with the unit.

This quite unequivocal response to the call for help had come with equal enthusiasm from the medical faculty of the university. Fifty-seven of its members were in the service of either the army or the navy, twenty of this number were in the University Base Hospital.

The loss of so many active staff members presented a serious problem. But the school was determined, as it has been determined in every similar situation since, that high-level preparation must go on without interruption.

It was perhaps fortunate for Miss Powell, in a stern, backhanded, backbreaking way, that she had had what amounted to a graduate course in making do. During the year of the United States' active participation in World War I, much was required of her, in a very great hurry and with no additional facilities at her command.

First, she had to fill the vacancies left by the nurses who had gone to army camps or overseas. For obvious reasons the substitutes were both less experienced and less physically strong than their predecessors had been. Yet it was necessary to ask more work of them than had been asked of the others. Only the sense of being deeply involved in a shared catastrophe could have kept the staff at a task which had always been arduous and which became, in 1917 and 1918, one for a feminine equivalent of Hercules. Miss Powell, probably in all her life, never spoke a sentimental or extravagant word (her reports are small masterpieces of restraint and understatement) but she was able nonetheless to inspire in her associates a sturdy conviction that this was a moment in which to demonstrate one's love of country instead of merely singing about it. Every one, she testified later, had responded with "fine courage and hearty cooperation."

Her second task was to accelerate the training program so that a stream of workers could be poured into the army camps if the war were to go on and on. The Committee of the School announced in 1917:

41

As a war measure college women with suitable scientific preparation will be admitted, subject to the usual requirements, for a two years' course of intensive study with the understanding that the required third year may be spent in war service in nursing and will entitle the nurse, so enlisting, to the usual degree.

In the event of the conclusion of the war before the two-year period of intensive study is completed the candidate for the degree will be expected to fulfill the third year of study in the University Hospital under the usual requirement for receiving the degree.

The war was not to be made an excuse for allowing standards to slip back into the old improvising ways. It might well be assumed that army assignments would supply a broad laboratory background for those who had seen actual service in camps or at the front. But a young woman must not hope to get a degree simply by putting on a uniform. She must still satisfy exacting requirements.

Miss Powell's third task was to become "acting superintendent" of the hospital. Dr. Baldwin had been borrowed, for the duration, by the surgeon general in Washington. This flattering acknowledgment of his success in implementing the base hospital took him to important work in national defense. But it left important work at home to be distributed among his associates. Miss Powell's letter, in response to that of President Marion LeRoy Burton, announcing her new appointment, said modestly that she hoped "with the cooperation of faculty and staff to be able at least to keep things going smoothly until Dr. Baldwin's return."

At the same time, in January, 1918, the assistant to the superintendent of the hospital went into uniform. Overnight, Miss Powell found that she had assumed the responsibilities of two men in addition to her own. For as acting superintendent of the hospital she did not cease to be superintendent of nurses. Nor did she cease to be the chief teacher in the school of nursing.

She simply gathered up all these tasks at once into her capacious apron.

Miss Powell's new appointment brought her into close association with a man who had vigorous ideas about what the education of the nurse should be.

Elias P. Lyon was before all else an educator. As a Ph.D. in physiology he had come to administration work by an unusual route, but his long career as dean of the medical school at Minnesota produced fine results for the profession. As Dr. Maurice Visscher has pointed out, "he believed firmly that no educational institution of quality can survive unless the members of its staff were imbued with the spirit of investigation. His determination to establish a group of medical teachers with such attitudes may be said, quite fairly, to be one of the most important reasons for the existence of the active medical research and teaching center in the University of Minnesota today."

Perhaps because he was not himself a doctor, Lyon had more flexibility than deans have sometimes shown in his relationship to the nurse and toward her work. Obviously he did not feel, as many another observer of the time did feel, that the nurse must be content forever to be merely another pair of hands for the doctor. It was Abraham Flexner who gave down the judgment that the nurse must be "like a sentinel in fresh energies [who] subordinates loyally her intelligence to his theory and policy and is effective in precise proportion to her ability to second his efforts."

With this traditional view Dean Lyon disagreed. He believed not merely in the ability of the nurse to play an active role in the care of the sick, but in her potential usefulness as a kind of "sub-doctor." But first, of course, her training would need to be lifted to a higher level of insight into the problems of science.

In an article, written in longhand and never published — perhaps because of controversial suggestions contained in it — Dean Lyon once pointed out that "good medical service" was not at the moment being made available to all the people of the United States; that the tendency of the family doctor to disappear had left "country places" seriously penalized by want of proper care; that to increase numbers by lowering standards would be a disaster for the profession; that it "might be better to provide a subordinate personnel within the reach of all people" and that highly trained graduate nurses might be licensed, after completing such an advanced course, as "Health Advisers" to serve rural communities "on a cooperative or community basis."

Since the idea never was pressed by Dean Lyon himself it would be improper to attempt to appraise its value in the light of present-day conditions. But what remains important is simply the fact that an influential man of science believed unreservedly in the potential usefulness of the nurse and that he played a significant part in developing a positive role for her to play. As he saw the sisterhood:

43

The nurses of the country have at least some training in the basic principles of medicine, obtained under medical men and in surroundings where good medicine is practiced. The nurses are accustomed to work with and under the direction of medical men. The nurses are socially minded, are not bound by traditions of economic theory, have an abiding interest in public health and consider education one of their primary functions.

The nurse has knowledge of treatment procedures and is skilled in the care of the patient. Her curriculum has given her training in the observation of disease . . . She tends to take the place in the home of the family physician. She is really the sub-doctor of the present age.

Believing that the nurse should be taught to fill that job more effectively, Dean Lyon cooperated closely with the advisory committee of the nursing school in planning courses to be taught by members of the medical faculty. It cannot have happened often in the teens of the century that nursing education had so many conscientious friends all in one place. Dean Lyon was a convinced supporter of its rights. Miss Powell, as acting superintendent of the hospital, was in attendance at all meetings of the administrative board of the medical school and could get its ear easily. Dr. Beard, as secretary of the medical school, could anticipate or support Miss Powell's suggestions.

A new triumvirate had been established.

Day after day the war created new crises. One was met by persuading Miss Pierce to return to Minnesota and take over some of Miss Powell's teaching duties. Despite the fact that many had done much to draw the nursing school close into the university system, in the view of some it still occupied a distant, not quite visible outpost on the educational frontier. Miss Pierce's salary was modest — $100 a month — but even this sum could not be found in the budget and had to be guaranteed by a private citizen.

The psychological crisis of the nurse who felt that experience had completely passed her by when she found herself unable to go overseas was solved by circumstance. Instead of the women in the School for Nurses having to seek out a war, war came to them.

It came in the very active persons of young hospital corpsmen, detailed by the United States Navy for instruction in medical services. They brought from Mare Island and Goat Island where they had been based all the sprightliness suggested by these names, and it was the job

44

of the school to transform them into nurses for hospital ships of the navy, the *Comfort*, the *Solace*, and the *Mercy*.

Washington had had the subversive idea of putting on board these ships expert surgical nurses. "What! Women on board!" groaned Admiral Goldbraid himself when he heard of the suggestion. A compromise had to be found. It consisted of calling the University of Minnesota once more into special service.

Commander Warren J. Terhune, U.S.N., visited the School for Nurses to ask what a landbound institution could offer his bluejackets. Miss Vannier, acting for Miss Powell, showed the outline of the course given to students in the preparatory course. It was, said the commander, precisely what was wanted if only it could be crowded into the four months that was to be allowed for instruction. Anything, Miss Vannier said in effect, can be condensed if sufficient heat is applied to it.

Her plan was to escort fifty men at a time into the operating room amphitheater where she would demonstrate the technique of one nursing process after another and describe the therapeutic value of each treatment or service. At the first session she met the corpsmen with dread, fearing that they would hate having to do women's work and hate her for having to teach them. Simply to try out her own voice and get it under control, she decided to call the roll. When only three names had been called, one sailor, into whose mind habit had bitten particularly deep, answered: "Here, sir." The idea of a delicate woman's being greeted like a stern old tar pleased everyone so much that an *entente cordiale* was immediately established between Miss Vannier and her strenuous charges.

After each lecture the men went, in sections of twenty, to classrooms for actual practice. Ten men were put to bed while ten others performed such actual procedures as making a bed with the patient in it. At first this seemed like an inexpensive but reasonably lively entertainment. But gradually the men became genuinely interested in their tasks. In the men's ward patients gladly volunteered to serve as practical material after Miss Vannier had explained to them that this was their contribution to the war effort.

The whole university system was drawn into the experiment. The medical school offered intensive theoretical instruction in bacteriology, physiology, minor surgery, and anatomy (with weekly sessions of dissection). The school of dentistry gave the young men a background in oral

45

hygiene. The College of Pharmacy introduced them to the study of pharmaceutical chemistry. Deans of these divisions often gave the lectures themselves.

But it was still the School for Nurses that assumed the greatest responsibility for this hasty induction into a knowledge of the healing arts. Miss Powell stole from the hospital six periods, an hour and a half each, to tell all that anyone could ever communicate about bandaging. Miss Pierce and student nurses who had already been through the course opened the way to understanding of such professional mysteries as "lavage, gavage and irrigation of eye, nose and throat . . . use of the Priessnitz compress . . . preparation for venesection . . . application of abdominal binders."

Miss Gertrude Thomas, dietitian, taught the young sailors the essentials of cookery for invalids "with emphasis on an understanding of food classifications, caloric values and the chemical digestion of nutrients." Each man had his stove, utensils, and ingredients with which to produce meals for the sick.

Obviously this was no hastily improvised pattern of instruction but a genuine experiment which could have been successful only in an institution that was experienced in the techniques of teaching. As the naval officer in charge of the men later reported in the *American Journal of Nursing*: "The method of individual instruction was made possible by [the university's] abundant facilities."

Miss Powell, herself well aware that the best way to learn is to teach, felt that the experience of catching a swarm of bluejackets and turning them into qualified pharmacist's mates had been invaluable to her students. The navy continued to send group after group far inland to Minnesota for the same instruction. A first detachment of one hundred men completed the work in January, 1918, to serve "somewhere on the Atlantic coast or at sea." A second hundred men were trained and ready for duty in May, when a third followed them promptly into Elliot Hospital.

This was the first coeducation that had been conducted within the School of Nursing. (It was not until after World War II — in 1949 — that men asked for formal admission as students and got it.) At first the accidental recruits of 1917 seemed to the women nursing students like aliens and interlopers. The best that could be said of them was that they were "nice boys" with their minds chiefly on the problems of organizing dances; the worst, that they were just "a bunch of crazy kids, glad to be away from home." The war seemed still to be rather pleasantly fantastic and unreal. The corpsmen could not immediately subdue their natural exuberance and "wanted to give anesthetics and assist with operations" on their first day in the hospital.

But gradually the attitude changed. The young men learned a great deal and when the war was over many of the three hundred returned to Minnesota to tell of their experiences, some of them to enroll as students of medicine and dentistry.

The experience of one, in particular, deserves to be recorded at length.

He had been stationed at the big navy base at Queenstown, Ireland, during the first big flu epidemic. The emergency was great and in the course of it many died. One night a navy doctor came to the ward and asked:

"Is there anyone here who knows how to give a sponge bath to reduce temperature?"

A Minnesota-trained pharmacist's mate stepped forward.

The patient was a high-ranking naval officer and it was apparent that he must die if relief for his condition were not provided quickly.

Said the young man afterward:

I made up my mind that this would be done right. I got out my notebook and read the procedure through. Then I put an ice cap on the patient's head and a hot water bag at his feet, placing him on a rubber sheet covered by a muslin sheet. I took his temperature and recorded it on the chart: brought in a basin of cold water and two sponges: began the bath using long smooth regular strokes, following the course of the large blood vessels, from the jugular vein under the ear. Right side of the neck . . . down right side of the body and leg to foot . . . turned the sponge and repeated the stroke. Continued on the right side for ten minutes . . . then drew the sheet over the right side and exposed the left, repeating the same process for ten minutes. Turned the patient on his side and sponged the back for ten minutes. Packed the patient in wet sheets and after ten minutes took the temperature and recorded it. There had been a satisfactory drop. In half an hour the doctor returned and looked at the chart, shook his head and asked for a thermometer. After taking the temperature and finding it still lower, he looked at me and asked: "What did you to do that man?" I drew myself up and said: "Sir, I gave him a University of Minnesota sponge."

The satisfactory epilogue to the story was that the corpsman was put in charge of teaching the entire group at the Queenstown base hospital.

47

At home in Minnesota the flu epidemic was also running wild. The disease, caused by an infection known as hemolytic streptococcus, produced a rupture of the red blood cells and allowed free blood to escape into the tissues; it was of demoralizing virulence.

Starting in the army camps of the Boston area it had swept down the Atlantic coast and then moved westward across the continent. By September, 1918, it had encircled and overwhelmed the Midwest. The civilian population was struck as violently as the men of the services had been, and the board of regents at the university voted to turn Elliot Hospital over to public service. It was emptied of all other patients and for eight weeks only influenza and pneumonia victims were admitted.

With all the experienced staff gone to war, the burden of this crisis fell on student nurses and medical internes. Overnight these young people were transformed from beginners into agents of the life force itself, required by the emergency to hold off death, if they could, by their own inner strength and to pretend, the while, to indestructibility. Eight hours constituted the regular day devoted to practice in the hospital but during the epidemic student nurses worked ten hours and, at night, often much longer. But this active service was only the beginning of their responsibility. The forenoon was usually spent in writing reports, after which they permitted themselves a few hours sleep and went back to the job. One student nurse, who had caught the disease early and made a quick recovery, returned to the wards and was regarded thereafter as the very embodiment of the will to confront danger. She worked virtually around the clock.

Conditions were appalling. Many patients were either dead or moribund upon arrival at the hospital and the tragic chorus of grief-stricken relatives echoed up and down the corridors. For pregnant women the diagnosis of flu was often equivalent to a death sentence. On the fourth floor, where these victims were concentrated, the lungs of three or four filled up each night and there was time to do no more than to wheel their bodies into the corridor, put a screen around them, and make way for the next patients.

It was in this moment that the men of the navy training school matured as members of an advanced course in human need. Commander Terhune sent groups of them to the hospital for four hours each day. The initiation of the apprentices was complete and many reported later that, grim as these experiences had been, they had served to make their

actual war service better than it might otherwise have been. For everyone who was deeply involved in this experience, the final effect was to
produce an unusually deep maturity of temper. A dozen students of that
day were to testify, by high achievement in their fields, that even disaster
and death can be teachers.

One of these students was Pearl L. McIver, later to be chief of the
Division of Public Health Nursing of the United States Public Health
Service.

In 1918 she was a junior student at Minnesota and her work was, at
the moment of the flu epidemic, in pediatrics. In a ward on the top floor
of the hospital, which ordinarily housed fifteen to twenty patients, she
had thirty children under her care, all night long, alone. These patients,
varying in age from two to ten, were desperately sick. Many had been
picked up by the police who found them in homes where the parents
already lay dead. Exhausted and frightened, they were bundled into
paddy wagons and carried to the hospital where they were met, in the
pediatrics ward, by creatures who frightened them still more.

The rules of the hospital required all personnel to wear masks, close-
fitting caps, and white gowns. This costume was supposed to protect
them against the disease; it did not do so.

On the first night when Miss McIver reported for duty, the day staff
was still in the ward. It seemed inhuman to leave one inexperienced girl
in a room where all the children were screaming in terror at the ghosts
that flitted about them. Every one of them was standing in his crib,
giving shrill voice to his terror of the unfamiliar and the unpredictable.
An already exhausted day nurse volunteered to stay on for the night as
well. But a subversive idea was at work in the mind of a young leader-
in-the-making, and Miss McIver begged to be left alone.

As soon as the last nurse had gone she pulled off the mask and cap
and restored herself to the status of a human being. Then one by one
she picked up each child in his own blanket and offered the reassurance
of normal tenderness. By some miracle of inadvertence there was an old
white rocking chair in a corner of the ward. With a child in her arms,
Miss McIver sat in that chair and rocked, knowing that she defied the
rules and the doctrine of the time which forbade picking up any occupant of the ward, at any time, for reasons other than those of strict
procedure. There was to be no coddling, let alone — sinister word! —
cuddling.

49

Yet very soon the children were asleep. Something quite normal had happened to them and they responded, in their exhaustion, by behaving normally. Then, as one by one they woke again, the nurse picked them up again and "forced fluids, the most important item in the treatment regimen."

On the fourth night of this private revolution, Miss McIver was caught in her subversive activity. An interne walked into the ward and looked on in utter incredulity. "What on earth are you doing?" he was able to ask at last. The end of her career had come, the nurse was sure; but she stood and faced the supposed enemy. "The children were scared stiff," she said. "I'm merely trying to make them feel comfortable and at home." After a moment the interne said quietly: "Have you a second rocking chair?"

Thereafter, they rocked together, night after night, sharing their guilt in gratifying defiance of the law. There was just one complication. Miss McIver had to record the fluid intake of her patients and the children took so much more liquid at night than they did during the day that eyebrows were raised and there was talk of padding the record. But neither she nor the interne ever told their secret.

Thirty years later, Miss McIver, then in government service in Washington, met a distinguished pediatrician who looked curiously familiar. He was the interne of the rocking chair. "The only trouble with you and me was," he said, "that we were twenty years ahead of our time."

While this exacting apprenticeship proceeded, the nurses continued to endure the primitive living conditions against which Miss Powell unavailingly protested. As new quarters were added to make room for the growing enrollment, these were still of the old kind, hastily remodeled family dwellings, old, flimsy, and hard to heat. The young women slept two to a room, and in winter, two to a bed so that double quantities of bedding could guard a little against the cold.

Youth saw them through these trials unfailingly. Survivors do not remember having experienced any bitterness of spirit. The young women had all the homely solaces of the undemanding: a swing on the front porch for use in summer; a telephone on the stair landing for use at all times through which every nurse could engage in vicarious flirtations with all the male friends of all the other girls in the household; bicycles which it gave them a now-inexplicable satisfaction to ride indoors from room to room. They gave pet names to the cockroaches in the kitchen sink and even regarded the rats as nothing worse than an undesirable minority. One girl who had joined a sorority returned from occasional visits to the comparative grandeur of the Kappa house with no feeling that she made a "descent to Avernus."

What pleased them most was the feeling that they were no longer aliens on the campus. When the first class of nurses had been presented at commencement to the president of the university, one of them had overheard a man from the School of Dentistry, seated just behind her, exclaim in disgust: "Well, what won't they graduate!" But after World War I this snobbery disappeared. As Miss Vannier once reported:

The student nurses wore the university colors [maroon and gold] in their nice warm capes. When a group of them crossed the campus to classes they made a pleasing splash of color against the snow and, because of their attractive appearance they were never forgotten, always included in university functions. This sometimes created a problem as it was not easy to excuse them from duty. But we were glad they were so popular and did all we could to cooperate.

In short, they belonged.

4

The Oneness of Our Common Lot

THE period of seven years from 1917 to 1924 was one of convulsive change for the United States and for the institutions which were asked to support its new position as a world power. During the war years the University of Minnesota had transformed itself from a campus into a camp. The School for Nurses was not the only one of its units that had taken on the look of military discipline. The College of Science, Literature, and the Arts had become the setting for an ill-starred experiment in trying to combine academic interests with those of a nation preparing for what might be a long struggle overseas. The sleepy young soldiers of the Students Army Training Corps, exhausted by drill in the city streets of Minneapolis, were marched into classrooms to sit, in a condition of utter bewilderment, through what were to them unintelligible discussions of Spenser's style and tedious examinations of the viscera of frogs. A conscientious, but badly considered, effort had threatened, as Minnesota educators said bluntly, to disrupt standards for a long time to come.

At the start of the national crisis, George Edgar Vincent had resigned to become president of the Rockefeller Foundation. To his place came Marion LeRoy Burton, red of hair and energetic of disposition. Through the whole of his short administration (1917 to 1920) he struggled with the exhausting problems of war and its aftermath. The university was in quite desperate need of an adequate physical plant and Burton's building program was both ambitious and imaginative. But before it was well started he, too, resigned to go to the University of Michigan. His successor, Lotus Delta Coffman, previously dean of the

College of Education at Minnesota, took up the unfinished tasks of creating a new campus and at the same time of restoring academic order.

He came to the presidency in an unhappy hour. The state of Minnesota was being given a preview of the depression which was presently to become worldwide. The whole agricultural community lay in the shadow of acute emergency and the state legislature lacked funds with which to support new enterprises or even to maintain old ones securely.

Yet, despite these difficulties, the period was one of enormous growth for the university both in numbers and in prestige. Coffman's qualities of leadership were distinguished and he put them, with impartial energy, at the service of every unit within the educational system.

During these years the School for Nurses was able to make three important contributions to the history of nursing education. The most significant of these advances was the establishment at Minnesota of one of the first five-year programs leading to the degree of bachelor of science.

This was the culmination of a long campaign on the part of the advisory committee to lift its pattern of instruction for the nurse to what was really the collegiate level. In 1912, the board of regents had given the ruling that graduates of the school were to receive what their resolution called "degrees." But this troubled Miss Powell's conscience because she could not believe that the education given her students was, in fact, equivalent to the education given men and women in the four-year program of the arts college for completion of which they received the bachelor's degree. To be sure, nurse students were required to satisfy the university's entrance standards and they were taught by university teachers, but in other respects their training resembled that of the traditional schools. Emphasis was still heavy on practical service in the hospital, much lighter than the committee would have it on theoretical classroom instruction. Miss Powell had agreed reluctantly that "putting the School for Nurses in the same class with other technical departments was a wise thing to do at the time." But she and her advisers waited eagerly for an opportunity to advance standards farther so that a degree from the School for Nurses should be earned by a discipline as exacting as that of any other college of the university system.

In June, 1919, she and her associates announced that they "felt prepared" to offer a course which combined work "pursued in the College of Science, Literature, and the Arts with work done in the School for Nurses." This "degree program" was designed to give the student a general education plus professional training. Its distinctive feature was that it required an applicant to have earned seventy-five university credits before she matriculated in the School.

The general design of courses to be followed throughout the five-year program was established by the committee of the school. But during her first two years the prospective nurse entered classes in the arts college and received instruction along with its own freshmen and sophomores. Studies in composition, English, zoology, psychology, chemistry, history, political science, and economics were designed to give her a background of liberal education against which the later clinical training of the nurse could be made more meaningful than it would otherwise have been.

Only after successful completion of five quarters devoted to this introductory study was the student nurse admitted to the school. For the following ten quarters she was in residence there and followed the basic professional sequence which constituted the major of the curriculum leading to the B.S. degree. The work of the ensuing three quarters consisted of electives designed to prepare teachers or public health nurses. Commencement day brought the student nurse a kind of dual recognition. Along with her academic degree she received the professional degree of graduate in nursing.

The degree program did not supplant the three-year program. The great majority of the school's students were still enrolled in it. Indeed, it would have been impossible to do without the matriculants in the diploma program. Society needed nurses and the school needed students quite as much as ever. In the first years of its existence the B.S. program attracted few applicants. Only two of seven who enrolled in 1919 stayed to complete the course and only twelve women were graduated from it in its first five years. The vital energy needed for survival of the first university school of nursing continued to come from the three-year students. Many years were to pass before another major change in tradition made it possible to drop the diploma program.

But the purpose of the school's creating the eighteen-quarter curriculum had been to strengthen nursing education at its base so that it might begin to produce the kind of leaders who were needed by the profession. The significant fact is that from the numerically small number of early graduates of Minnesota's degree program came many of the professional workers who, during the next quarter of a century, were to distinguish themselves in nursing organizations, in other schools, in public health

54

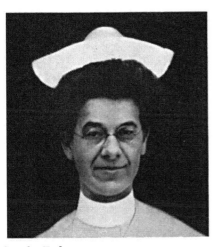

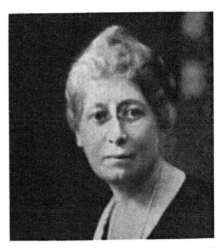

Bertha Erdmann
director 1909–1910

Louise M. Powell
director 1910–1924

*Former directors of the School of Nursing at the
University of Minnesota*

Marion Vannier
director 1924–1930

Katharine J. Densford
director 1930–1959

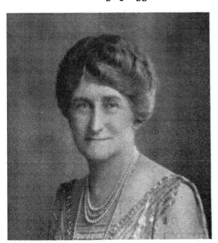

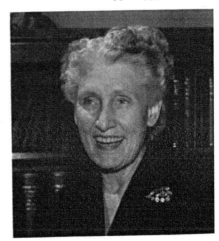

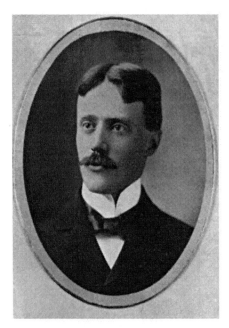

Dr. Louis Baldwin, re-designer of
the University's hospital facilities

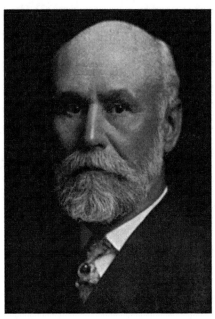

Richard Olding Beard, "Nestor
of Nurses"

Elias P. Lyon, influential early dean
of the Medical School

Harold S. Diehl, dean of the
Medical School 1935–1958

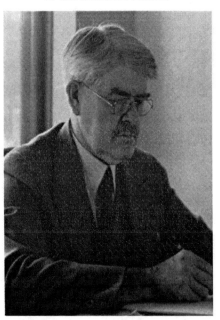

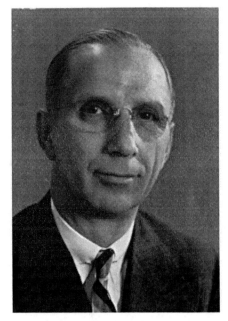

activities all over the nation, and also in this country's contribution to the health programs of foreign lands.

As though to mark a break with the past the school changed its name. On April 14, 1920, the board of regents authorized the new look. Gone was the School for Nurses, a designation to which there clung some hint of the old apprentice system of instruction, and in its place the School of Nursing emerged, declaring more appropriately a chief concern with the subject matter of nursing education.

The second contribution made to nursing history during the crowded years of the 1920's was the creation of the so-called Central School.

For many years the National League of Nursing Education had been preaching the doctrine that three things must be done to improve the training of the nurse. Schools must deepen the content of instruction, broaden the field of the student's experience, and unify procedures of preparation. All that had been hit or miss in the fortunate or unfortunate practices of the past must be brought under the discipline of one high standard. Unification became the important word.

Dean Lyon became convinced that the best way to accomplish all these aims at once would be to establish, in his own community, one large, important center of nursing education. Minnesota medicine had done the same thing for itself when Dr. Millard had managed to unify instruction for physicians in one strong school at the university instead of allowing it to be scattered through many schools with differing standards of responsibility. Why, he wondered, should there not be a similar central school for nurses?

In February, 1920, he offered his idea to Dr. Walter List, superintendent of the Minneapolis General Hospital. He wrote:

The nurse needs a background of chemistry, anatomy and physiology for exactly the same reasons that the doctor needs this background. It is to be obtained in exactly the same place and under the same conditions as in the case of the doctor; that is, in a good school, with good laboratories and good teachers. Such facilities are found in universities. They are not likely to be found in hospitals.

I should like to see *one* school of nurses in Minneapolis, just as there is one medical school. I should like to see strong, appropriate and adequate fundamental courses developed in the university for all nurses of the city. From these courses I should like to see the candidates go to the various hospitals for their practical training still under unified supervision and with such methods of transfer and instruction as would ensure an all-around training for all. I should like to see all candidates finally examined and graduated by the university, the state's best mechanism for standardization and certification in educational matters.

This is a vision to be realized only by time and evolution. But it will not realize itself. Those who hold the vision must work for it.

It was much less hard than Dean Lyon had supposed it would be to persuade a man of Dr. List's drive and imagination to try an experiment. In the fall of 1920 he sent four women who had applied for training in his hospital to do preparatory work at the university. The results pleased both the students and the supervisors in charge of their work when they returned to the Minneapolis General. As everyone agreed, they entered the practical phase of training with a better understanding of objectives than was usual among beginners. On the basis of this experience the Minneapolis General offered formally, in December, 1920, to give up its own school, renounce all training activities and accept as its students women enrolled in the School of Nursing at the university.

The exigencies of the moment were involved in Dr. List's decision. He was concerned chiefly with the fact that there had been a shortage of applicants for his own school. The promise of a standardized system of preparation such as the university could offer might, he hoped, attract more.

From Miss Powell's point of view the advantages of this kind of affiliation were obvious. She had always been troubled by the fact that, at Elliot Hospital, student nurses had only limited opportunity to study maternity cases, pediatric cases, and cases of contagious disease. At Minneapolis General a much broader field of study was opened.

With another institution of the Twin Cities the university hospital and the School of Nursing had close links. The recently established Charles T. Miller Hospital in St. Paul had just borrowed Dr. Baldwin, on a part-time basis, to plan and supervise its opening. With him had gone Miss Vannier, on loan, to organize the nursing service. This mutual dependence having been comfortably established between the university world and the directors of the Miller Hospital, it was inevitable that the new institution should look favorably on Dean Lyon's plan. The clinical range of the Miller was strictly limited and the directors did not want to start a school of their own. If the university were to supervise the training of its student nurses a wasteful duplication of effort could be avoided.

Again, as the committee of the university school saw readily, advantages worked both ways. At Miller Hospital students would see private patients, an experience which the university hospital could not offer them.

Two important institutions of the Twin Cities were now ready to participate in a cooperative experiment and the impulse toward unification of nursing education took on almost the look of a parade. The Northern Pacific Beneficial Association Hospital, operated by a fraternal organization of railroad employees, asked also to become a participant in the plan if it were to be activated.

On February 26, 1921, just a year after Dean Lyon had offered his suggestion to Dr. List, representatives of the several hospitals met with him and Dr. Beard to formulate a general policy. They agreed readily on essential details. Applicants must have earned high school diplomas; they must be twenty years old (later the age limit was reduced to eighteen); they must pass a physical examination; they must complete a preliminary course successfully; they must pay a forty-dollar tuition fee. The university was to provide housing the cost of which would be paid, on a pro rata basis, by the several outside hospitals and by the university hospital.

The plan proposed that at the end of the preliminary course successful candidates for diplomas should be assigned to the various hospitals of the group; each institution would receive a share "according to its need." Students who had maintained averages of A or B during the preliminary course might have first choice of what were to be their "home hospitals." Others took the assignments given them by the school committee. Soon, however, a certain percentage of students from each letter-grade category was sent to each hospital. But by a system of rotation each nurse student must go, at some period, to each hospital so that she might have the benefit of the wide field experience that the group had to offer. And, as Dean Lyon had suggested originally, the student was to receive her diploma at last as graduate of the university.

This was the outline of the work of the Central School, as the participants agreed to call it. No formal contract was ever signed by the representatives of the hospitals, but a memorandum of agreement was drawn up and agreed upon. By vote of the board of regents in March, 1921, the Central School became a reality.

It would seem to be a constant feature of the history of experimentation that moments of fresh inspiration coincide with moments of the greatest awkwardness for the administrative sponsors of new ideas. Dean Lyon and Dr. Beard promptly learned that the Central School had come into existence in just such a difficult time.

During 1921 the shadows of the agricultural depression steadily deepened. The legislature, meeting in that year, was "troubled by many things" and it tended to look severely down its collective nose at any hint of extravagance. A legislative committee slashed the president's budget for the university into ribbons, leaving Coffman in the gravest doubt as to how the fragments were to be drawn together to cover needs decently.

The whole community was astir with anxiety. A "Save the University" campaign among students added some unexpected and altogether creditable incidents to the history of loyalty to alma mater. Defenders rallied everywhere throughout the state. Within the legislature itself vigorous leaders rose to urge reconsideration of the problem. The demonstrations offered striking evidence of deep concern for the good of education.

But before the problems of the budget could be resolved, Dean Lyon and Dr. Beard were warned again and again that there must be no thought of additional expenditure in connection with plans for expansion of the School of Nursing. President Coffman, who was neither a patient man nor one who tended to minimize the schoolman's chronic fear of his institution's extinction, wrote that unless the legislature should unexpectedly turn generous the university would have to "sell supplies, equipment, live-stock and everything we can obtain to make up the budget."

One of his fears was that Miss Powell might now expect to leave her job as superintendent of nurses in the hospital and assume a new, more important role as director of the School of Nursing. That would not be possible in the circumstances as Dean Lyon felt obliged to point out with a quite uncharacteristic touch of severity. There would be no new titles, no new positions, just more responsibilities.

Miss Powell replied with the reserve of a woman who had long since learned that, in the midst of the whirlwind of a struggling institution's life, the poise of an administrator must remain unshaken. Any suggestion of expansion for the school, made by the committee, referred only to the future, she said, "when the larger school is beginning to prove itself a success." With admirable docility she continued to be superintendent of nurses in the hospital.

In the end President Coffman was not obliged to lead the cows to the block in a forced sale. The university was saved by the concerted efforts of faculty, students, and the public in general. With the dramatic effect of a last-minute reprieve, the legislature voted to restore many of the allowances that it had proposed to slash from the budget, and the university community returned from the dizzy heights of panic to the normal level of struggle.

For the School of Nursing this meant working within the old familiar pattern of improvisation toward justification of hopes for the Central School. Dr. Beard had observed in the *American Journal of Nursing* that Minnesota offered "an object lesson" in the development of a new and better kind of professional education. This pride of the explorer needed to be endorsed by practical achievements.

These were not long in revealing themselves. The training of the nurse steadily improved. No longer was she obliged to follow the deadening monotony of set routines. Instead she functioned in many different situations and had intimate views of every kind of experience. She could no longer have a limited outlook upon her profession.

Further, the atmosphere of the Central School was sympathetic to experimentation. Officials of the university worked with four different administrators in its own hospital, in the Minneapolis General, in the Miller, and in the Northern Pacific Hospital in St. Paul. If one of these administrators proved reluctant to try a new idea, another would be sure to seize upon it eagerly. It was no static society through which the student nurse made her way toward understanding, but one of vigorous movement and great variety.

Just six months after the Central School began to receive matriculants Miss Powell went on leave to complete work for her own B.S. degree. Miss Vannier became acting superintendent of nurses in her place.

Her job of integrating all the interests of four institutions was intricate. A total of more than 1,250 beds had to be cared for in the course of the day's work and the occupants of those beds presented problems of every kind in the calendar of illness except the problems of psychopathology. Fortunately, the many people involved were able to work together harmoniously. The hospitals were all fully staffed and no disruptive rivalries developed. Indeed, the correspondence between the university and the affiliated institutions exposes not one prima donna of the kind often unmasked by intimate glimpses of projects that are hopefully called "cooperative."

When Miss Powell returned to Minnesota, in January, 1923, she made generous acknowledgment of what had been accomplished "by those who carried through the plan for the Central School." She was, she wrote, "amazed." And she may well have been for she faced a new world of responsibility. Already the experiment had begun to fulfill the aims which it was designed to reach. Not the least of these was the recruitment of more members for the uncrowded profession of nursing. The contribution made by the Central School was significant. In the academic year 1923–24, its enrollment doubled. Miss Powell faced a student body of three hundred members.

A third achievement in which the School of Nursing had an honorable share was the creation of a course in public health work. This unit of the university system, which came to be known at last as the school of public health, developed through many phases, and under the usual number of academic aliases. It began as protégé of the medical school. But to the end of her life Miss Powell continued to take satisfaction in the fact that "this fine course drew its first breath in the School of Nursing."

Almost as soon as he had come to Minnesota Dean Lyon had begun to disturb the consciences of his colleagues about the need for a public health service. In his 1914 report to the president of the university the dean observed apologetically that it had proved to be "impossible to activate this division as a teaching unit." He was even more distressed in 1917 to have to acknowledge that the university still "made a poor showing" in matters related to safeguards against disease. Though the university hospital was supposed to "serve the needy of the state," little was being done in the field of preventive medicine. With the "prompt cooperation of the State Board of Health" cases of infectious disease were "handled on the whole successfully." But dispensary and infirmary were "wholly absent." The responsibility owed by a public institution to its community was being miserably neglected.

A first step toward repair of the situation which so troubled Dean Lyon's conscience was made in the summer of 1918. A member of the hospital staff was assigned to the task of working with the Minnesota Public Health Association to design a course for teachers and workers in the field of public health. This was the "first breath" of which Miss Powell spoke, drawn by a nurse of her organization and imparted, precariously at first, to a slight infant destined to grow into one of the most distinguished schools of its kind in the country.

Dorothy Slade Kurtzman set about the job of creating the university's first course in public health with both the courage and the uncertainty of the pioneer. It is indicative of the conditions under which an innovator worked in the early part of the century that it was considered magnanimous to relieve her of all nursing duty for the period spent in inventing something quite new.

Though her association with the university had been of long standing, Mrs. Kurtzman had begun as neither nurse nor teacher. In the days when President Vincent was developing his idea of the "statewide university" by sending out Chautauqua groups of faculty members and others to carry the atmosphere of the classroom into the towns of Minnesota, Mrs. Kurtzman had shared in the experiment. Having then no thought of nursing as a career she had prepared for one as an entertainer. Reading the poems of Browning and Tennyson to audiences of farmers and their wives during "University Week" she had learned much about the Chautauqua system. Later she took her degree as graduate in nursing at the university and began a long career in its service, as superintendent of nurses.

Despite the unusual breadth of her background, Mrs. Kurtzman was modestly doubtful of her ability to put together a pattern of instruction the like of which had not existed in her days as a student. There were few precedents to follow and no textbooks to serve as guides. It was necessary for her and her associates to organize principles as they went along, depending largely on the practical wisdom of active workers in public health agencies.

Relying in part on her experience of the early days with President Vincent on the Chautauqua tours, she brought together the best lecturers in the field whom the community could supply. All of these co-workers were conscientious and able; some were brilliant. The most conspicuous, perhaps, was Dr. Mabel Ulrich, whose subject was social hygiene. This gifted graduate of the medical school at the Johns Hopkins University set a high standard. The composite of Dr. Ulrich's physical features and qualities of mind — red hair, challenging eyes, witty tongue, and incisive directness — made her a compelling figure on the platform. Using her wit as a whip against sham and inertia, she swooped and soared over the whole field of ideas, stimulating awareness of human need. Whether she was concerned, as in her early years, with health and public welfare or, as in her later activities, with books and criticism, Dr. Ulrich was always a powerful influence. Her contribution to the university's first course in public health offered a model of insight into essential problems. This beginning was modest and, by present-day standards, limited in scope. It consisted only of a four-month schedule devoted to discussions of social hygiene, rural nursing, and visiting nursing. Its distinction lay in the fact that it established a foundation on which the broad and significant work of later years could be built.

Then, suddenly, just as the first lectures in this series were being offered in November, 1918, the flu epidemic swept over the nation, grimly emphasizing the importance of preventive medicine. The movement to safeguard health before disease could seize disastrous command took on the compulsive strength of dread. As one public official said at the time: "We do not know much about what caused this disease; but we do know one thing; it must not happen again."

All circumstances conspired to make the development in public health work swift and vigorous. Nurses returning to civilian duty after the war years were looking for new and important work to do. The conservation of health as a national asset became a part of the program of government. The desire to make sure that the flu epidemic did not happen again seized upon the imagination of leaders everywhere. As Dr. C. E. A. Winslow of Yale observed, "the untilled fields of public health must have the best energies of well-trained men and women."

As president of the Rockefeller Foundation, George Edgar Vincent sponsored a survey of nursing education which underscored the need for an army of workers to carry the public health job far "beyond its earlier objectives of community sanitation and control of contact diseases by the use of sera and vaccines." What the country needed was a campaign of public education, one that would spread the gospel of controlling disease.

In this atmosphere of concern for fundamental problems of human well-being the University of Minnesota gradually evolved its own program. Since 1919 Dr. John Sundwall, professor of hygiene and director of the University Health Service, had been working toward the development of a department dealing with health. On April 26, 1922, such a unit was officially established in the medical school. In various phases it bore various names. Long known as the department of preventive medicine and public health, it became, after World War II, the School of Public Health. At the time of its creation Dr. Harold S. Diehl became its head. As successor to Dr. Sundwall he became director also of the Health Service.

This marked the beginning of a distinguished career. Dr. Diehl was graduated from the university's medical school in 1918. Both his alma mater and the nation as a whole were presently to receive abundant evidence of his ability to serve the work of public health.

The School of Nursing continued to work in close cooperation with Dr. Diehl's department. But besides this academic partnership there were other influences which made the link intimate. Through its graduates the school made important contributions to the history of the rapidly growing younger unit. These young women embodied the impulse to serve what Dean Lyon had called "the vital entity of science." They helped to draw into one continuing progress report all of Minnesota's enterprises in the health field.

The class which Miss Powell presented to the president in 1919 was make up of strikingly able women. The moment seemed to be one in which distinction became contagious. Many members of that group reached high place in public work. Among them were Anna Jones (later Mrs. E. S. Mariette), Hortense Hilbert (later Mrs. Nicholas Cikovsky), Alma Haupt, and Pearl McIver. Recognizing their unusual abilities, Miss Powell arranged for the first three to spend a year in post-graduate work at the Johns Hopkins Hospital School of Nursing. They were chosen partly because all had entered the School for Nurses with college degrees and had, therefore, a broader background than was usual. All of them presently returned to Minnesota to enter public health work on the local scene before moving on to play conspicuous roles in dramatizing what the Rockefeller Report called "the oneness of our common lot." Anna Jones Mariette and Alma Haupt were intimately concerned with the job of helping Dr. Diehl and his chief assistant, Dr. Ruth Boynton, to develop courses for their department. They first taught such things as Field Practices in Infant Welfare and Practice in County Nursing; the second, Mental Hygiene and Field Service in Visiting Nursing.

Highly individual and spirited as these two women were, their personal histories showed a curious similarity of background. A cluster of like influences produced in each the same preoccupation with social responsibility. Mrs. Mariette was the descendant of a long line of leaders in the business and cultural life of Minneapolis; Alma Haupt came of an equally long and useful line of citizens prominent in the religious and cultural life of St. Paul. Mrs. Mariette was graduated from Smith in 1915; Miss Haupt from the arts college at Minnesota in the same year. They entered the School for Nurses in 1916 and, for forty years thereafter, were uninterruptedly occupied with the task of promoting human welfare through public health projects.

Alma Haupt went on many missions, the most important of which, perhaps, was that of director, for the Commonwealth Fund, of nursing in Austria after World War I. There she helped to reshape a war-shattered country by introducing for the first time, into its rural districts, American ideas of public service.

Mrs. Mariette was not only deeply concerned with the activities that made her husband a figure of international importance in the fight against tuberculosis but entered, quite on her own, into the job of mitigating misery in one crisis after another. During World War II some 1,800 volunteer nurses were trained under her guidance for Red Cross work. In the polio epidemics of the mid-1950's she organized emergency services.

If the first breath of life in the School of Public Health came from the School of Nursing the vital energies of many of its graduates were also imparted, freely and effectively, to the later phases of its development.

These three achievements — establishment of nursing education on a college level by the creation of the curriculum leading to the bachelor of science degree, standardizing the preparation of the nurse in Minnesota by bringing together the Central School, assisting significantly in the development of the School of Public Health — were the important developments in the history of the School of Nursing during World War I and after.

There were other signs of progress. In the academic year 1922–23, a course was created for instructors in schools of nursing. At the same time there began a long and close cooperation with the College of Education through a course designed for school nurses. Both of these were foreshadowings of the important work which the School of Nursing was later to do in the field of advanced study.

64

When Miss Powell returned from her leave in 1923 she found a greatly changed school. The financial troubles of the earlier 1920's had receded far enough so that the president could think — as he would always have wished to do — of educational advances rather than of budgetary retreats. Miss Powell was permitted, at last, to assume the title of director of the School of Nursing, and to devote her time to the job of administrator. To Miss Vannier went her old assignment as superintendent of nurses. University approval of what had been accomplished went to the ultimate extent of extending faculty rank not merely to the director but to superintendents, to their assistants, and to the teaching staffs of the affiliated hospitals.

Miss Powell moved with no pomp at all, yet with deep gratification, into offices in Millard Hall. There she presided over a minute staff. She had a full-time stenographer and a place to keep her records. In her office she met with members of the advisory committees. Of these there were now two. One was responsible for the policies of the school; the other made assignments of students to the hospitals. The dean of the medical school, the superintendents of the several hospitals, and the superintendents of nurses served with the director on the first; the superintendents of nurses served with the director on the second. Faithful Dr. Beard served on both.

It was a strikingly different world from the one into which Miss Powell had come a decade and a half earlier. The school had become part of the university system. It had complicated but well organized relationships with the colleges of medicine, dentistry, arts, and education. Its influence reached out across Minneapolis and St. Paul through the affiliated hospitals. It was looked upon neither as a curious whim on the part of "visionary educationists" nor as an inferior social agency. It represented a profession and it represented that profession well.

Miss Powell was not destined to enjoy for long the justification of her hopes. In 1924 she was persuaded to become dean of the Western Reserve University School of Nursing. But she never forgot Minnesota. Letters came from her regularly addressed with spontaneous empathy and with no sentimentality at all to "My dear children."

She, perhaps, regarded the school itself as no less her child. She had seen it through precarious infancy and anxiety-ridden childhood. As she left it she could feel that, rugged as its adolescence had been, there was the stuff of survival in it.

5

Ferment of Ideas

A PLACE where ideas are in ferment must always present a baffling kind of drama to the casual observer. A political arena, for example, in which champions of opposing attitudes slug heartily while they obviously entertain toward each other only the most friendly personal regard never seems quite real to the man who has no talent for fine, or for rugged, distinctions. But to the initiate there is a world of difference between the blow struck for truth and the blow struck for blood.

During the early 1920's when the university School of Nursing was strenuously engaged in pushing toward completion its plan for improved instruction in the affiliated hospitals, a mighty storm blew across the whole United States and tore the subject of nursing education wide open. It is not really a coincidence that three of the men most prominently involved were closely associated with the University of Minnesota. As a center of discussion, long since committed, indeed committed from its beginning, to a belief in the importance of the theoretical analysis of attitudes, the university was bound to be in the very midst of the ferment.

The three opponents were Dr. Charles Mayo, co-founder of the Mayo Clinic and friend of the university; George Edgar Vincent, president of the Rockefeller Foundation and former president of the university; and, of course, that indefatigable defender of his faith, Dr. Beard.

It was Dr. Charlie Mayo who brought the subject of education for the nurse to the attention of a large general public. In an authorized interview with a feature writer for the *Pictorial Review* he addressed himself briskly to a matter that could not fail to interest that magazine's following of women. Since the cost of care for the sick is still very much in the public mind an examination of the historical background of the argument continues to be of timely interest even today. It is of especial importance in a study of the development of the university's School of Nursing since theoretical considerations about education were involved.

Dr. Mayo began his statement with deliberately startling generalizations. "The nursing union," he said, "has become the most autocratic closed shop in the world." He did not "blame nurses for organizing." They had been driven to it by the "apparent deafness of those in authority" — their own leaders. But wages of $7 for an eight-hour day were "prohibitive." They denied "the divine right of care to the poor."

There were many important matters on Dr. Mayo's mind. The interview had much to say about "the public endowment of hospitals as instruments of public welfare" and about the establishment of "health centers in which girls of marriageable age might be taught effective home care of the sick." Though he was never a man who, as he himself liked to say, was given to making "balloon ascensions," he soared widely over the whole field — the past, the present, and the future — of nursing in the United States.

But the central and immediate point of what he had to suggest was that nurses were at the moment being overtrained. He said, "The educational standards for registration of nurses as set down by the nursing boards of the various states have gone beyond all reason. Any intelligent girl can acquire in two years all the knowledge necessary for the thoroughly competent nurse. I know that in my work I have never asked any nurse to do anything which she could not have learned how to do in two years' training."

What Dr. Mayo wanted — and in a hurry — was an army of young women trained in this less ambitious way. The title given to his interview was: "Wanted — 100,000 Girls for Sub-Nurses." It was curious that writer and editor should have clung stubbornly to this slightly sensational challenge. The body of the article explicitly repudiated its implications.

"For the sake of better emphasis," Dr. Mayo said, "I must revert to the sub-nurse. This is a title that does not sound good to my ears, for I think it is superfluous and unnecessary. The term nurse should be inclusive. The proper adjustment lies not in nurses and sub-nurses but in a modified, uniform law setting the standard at two years' high school education and two years' general hospital work. Then for the ambitious there could be special graduate courses in higher nursing."

It did not take Dr. Beard long to unlimber his fountain pen and shoot off sharp rejoinders in his most precise longhand. He and Dr. Mayo had long been associates in the conduct of the affairs of the university. They had been opponents in some issues over policy and allies in others. As to the importance of the contribution that had been made by the Mayo brothers to medical education, Dr. Beard had no doubt at all. He was the author of an article, published in 1914 by *Journal-Lancet*, which called attention to many of their services to the university. But now he felt that the position which he had worked so long to gain for nursing education was being undermined by a powerful force and he brought up his big guns of rhetoric to defend it.

So the two men squared off, not as personal enemies, but like two friends debating ideological differences in public. Just as he quite cheerfully put six lumps of sugar in his tea, in defiance of friends in the dental college who threatened him with the prompt decay of his teeth, he defied Dr. Charlie when his colleague threatened him with decay of nursing tradition through overblown standards of training. He was sure that neither calamity would occur.

Dr. Beard's answering article was long in getting into print. The editor of the *Pictorial Review*, feeling that the cream of public interest had been skimmed off, was reluctant to ply his readers with milk, however good it might be for them. Both Miss Nutting and Miss Isabel Stewart of Teachers College, Columbia, had to prod the conscience of the fourth estate before Dr. Beard's once-rejected article could be retrieved from the files and published.

By this time Dr. Mayo had been given the platform of the *American Journal of Nursing* from which to speak, this time directly to the profession. In a brief article, published in January, 1922, he restated his position with welcome clarification and even some hints of modification.

I do not advocate lowering standards, or shortening years of study: on the contrary I wish to make it possible for the nurse to attain a reputation by advancing standards through specialization . . . a two-year course of study combined with practical training in a hospital should be required for general nursing. An optional third year may be taken as a continuation of study or for special training in thousands of unfilled situations. Positions as school, city, county, industrial and welfare nurse, surgeons' assistants, dentists' assistants, hospital chief nurses, anesthetists, laboratory technicians represent but a few of the opportunities offered.

But he still believed that nurses had lowered the dignity of the profession by associating themselves with "carpenters, masons and plumbers" who sought to "control work and wages by unions and by limiting the number of apprentices in training." He reminded nurses that the "relief of the sick comes first" and, in a quotation from Woodrow Wilson, presented the challenge: "Do you covet distinction? You will get it only as the servant of mankind."

In the February issue of the magazine that started the controversy Dr. Beard returned to the forum. At almost the same moment, he put his ideas into expanded form and delivered them in person before the Central Council of Nursing Education, holding its annual meeting on January 30, 1922, at Chicago.

In that talk he described, with complete knowledge and no admiration, the way of the old-fashioned "institutional" school of nursing where "pupil nurses were exploited for the benefit of the hospitals." The length of the course was determined not by the students' needs but by the hospital's needs. The content of teaching, Dr. Beard said, was represented "by long, long hours of ward duty supplemented by a few crumbs of knowledge intermittently fed to pupils too weary to digest them."

Progessive ideas (like that represented by Minnesota's experiment with a university school) had just begun to bend men's minds toward the future when the war intervened to give "society at large and everywhere an awakened consciousness of the superlative value of human health. It created a growing demand for the public service of trained women to conserve these health values through a score of health agencies."

Dr. Beard went on to observe that society had begun to produce a new type of student upon whom "the evangel of service had taken hold." Unlike their predecessors in the field of nursing, these were capable of asking questions as well as of taking orders. And their chief questions were: "What is my job?" and "Am I fitted for the job?" As Dr. Beard, with his taste for apt quotation, permitted himself to imagine, they had begun to pray the prayer of Phillips Brooks, "not for tasks equal to their powers but for power equal to their tasks."

Next, he referred directly to the Mayo interview. The formula offered in it for the creation of the sub-nurse was, he believed, "the very reductio ad absurdum." These sub-nurses, as he interpreted Dr. Mayo's ideas were, "to be made out of country girls, financially unable to secure a high school education, accustomed to simple conditions of living, unpossessed of the spirit of social unrest but willing to work for a relatively small wage. And they are to be prepared for the business of subnursing, not by a sound education that would make them safe in the handling of human life, but by a brief course in the technique of a nurse's training."

Dr. Beard's central point was that such women simply could not do the work that the world had come to expect of nurses. If the movement toward higher education were to be choked off by economic limitations of the present moment, the enormous task of nurturing a healthy race for the future could not even be begun.

It seemed unreasonable to Dr. Beard to complain of a nurse's wage which was "not in excess of the cost of common or unskilled labor and far less than skilled labor even now secures." There was, to be sure, the problem of how to keep nursing care from being an intolerable burden to people in the middle income bracket. He said,

The obligation rests not upon the nursing profession alone but upon the nursing organizations, the relief agencies, upon our social bodies in general to get together for the solution of this grave problem.

To offer to the narrowly circumscribed an initially cheap, inexperienced untrained or inferior nurse is miserably to beg the question and inexcuseably to shirk a social duty. The wealthy can buy, at pleasure, the services of the graduate nurse. The indigent receives through grace of taxation the same quality of nursing care. The majority of our families who stand economically between these groups have a right to as good a quality of service. It is a matter of achieving the mechanism of supply and of educating the people to use it.

Dr. Beard could not, in the end, resist the temptation to match eloquence and sentiment with Dr. Mayo. The latter had said, "The good nurse is born. All the training in the world will not make a good nurse of a girl who is always thinking of herself and whose heart does not go out toward suffering humanity in a desire to ease that pain by self-sacrificing service." ("He might have said the same of the doctors or the members of any other profession or trade for that matter," said the New York Times on its editorial page, getting into the act just long enough to deflate Dr. Mayo's rarely used balloon.)

Dr. Beard may be thought to have done a balloon ascension, too, in his peroration but realistic insight balanced exalted sentiment neatly in his statement: "The nurse may be born in body, yet she needs none-theless the full values of educational training; but she whose devoted and disciplined spirit, with each new day of service is born again, is a nurse indeed."

There was one more chapter to be written into this animated dis-cussion of the nurse's education. It was inspired by the third man with a Minnesota background, Vincent of the Rockefeller Foundation. For three years a committee of the Foundation had been investigating nurs-ing schools of every kind. Under the secretaryship of Josephine Gold-mark (an extremely able analyst who was not influenced by any of the preoccupations that might have distracted a member of the profession from impartial appraisal), the wards and classrooms had been explored for the most minute details of procedure.

Miss Goldmark's findings were both encouraging and disturbing. The worst of them was that:

the average hospital school is not organized on such a basis as to con-form to the standards accepted in other educational fields; that the in-struction in such schools is frequently casual and uncorrelated; that the educational needs and health of the students are frequently sacri-ficed to practical hospital exigencies; that such shortcomings are pri-marily due to lack of independent endowment for nursing education; that existing educational facilities are on the whole, in the majority of schools, inadequate for the preparation of the high grade of nurses re-quired for all the rapidly accumulating tasks of the profession.

The best hope for the future lay in the development of the university schools of nursing. The report called their appearance in sixteen uni-versity centers "the most notable feature in the program of nursing education during the past ten years." Their strengthening was "of fun-damental importance in the furtherance of nursing education." From these university schools must come the superintendents, supervisors, in-structors, and public health nurses who were so urgently needed by all the communities of the United States.

With all this Dr. Beard was, of course, in hearty and grateful agree-ment. When the 500-page report of the Rockefeller Foundation ap-peared in 1923 it was found to contain many references to the School of Nursing at Minnesota as a "pioneer" in the advance of nursing edu-cation and as an institution which had continued, in all its movements of expansion, to offer an example for others to follow. But most reassur-ing of all else was the Rockefeller committee's conclusion that for the care of persons suffering from serious and acute disease the safety of the patient and the responsibility of the medical and nursing professions demand the maintenance of the standards of educational attainment now generally accepted by the best sentiment of both professions and embodied in the legislation of the more progressive states; and that any attempt to lower these standards would be fraught with danger to the public.

What Dr. Beard regarded as the most "vital observation" of the report was the comment that "It is the experience in every other field of education that the way to attract students is to raise the standards, not to lower them.

Yet in one of its findings the report gave more comfort to Dr. Mayo than to Dr. Beard. For it did recommend the encouragement of training for what it called "a subsidiary grade of nursing," one that might well prove to be sufficient in "the mild and chronic cases of convalescent care." To identify these "partially trained workers" the report avoided the term sub-nurses, calling them instead "nursing aides or attendants."

The Rockefeller report warned that there was danger "in the existence of a loosely defined and unregulated group of hospital workers" and that steps should be taken, through state legislation, not merely to establish standards of qualification but to provide for licensure. After that it would still be the job of the profession to make sure that training courses were provided for these nursing assistants. Instruction should be given "in appropriate places, under the strict supervision of the agencies governing the control of training schools for nurses themselves."

When he made his own "review and critique" of the Rockefeller Foundation report and read it before two different joint sessions of nursing organizations, Dr. Beard was still not reconciled to the idea of what he continued to call reproachfully the sub-nurse.

The committee's own belief, as he pointed out, was that such a new type of nursing service would not affect the economic problem greatly. "Sub-nurses" could not be expected to accept "a salary level much below that of the registered nurses." The scale was already low enough so that a significant reduction would be to depress earnings to a sub-subsistence level.

Dr. Beard held staunchly to the opinion that "the sub-nurse with her store of little knowledge will be dangerous because she does not know the end of her tether. No tag will efficiently label her. No law will keep her within safe bounds. No economy will be realized."

72

But he wasn't really worried. He offered as his final word the suggestion that "If we make the graduate nurse, and the public health nurse and the nursing educator and the institutional nurse educationally what they ought to be — society will find neither room nor need for any other and lesser type."

It remained for Vincent to conclude the discussion with a nod toward Dr. Mayo on his right and Dr. Beard on his left and to offer an endorsement of professional pride and ambition that would satisfy each. He wrote,

To both medical education and public health work the modern trained nurse is indispensable. For the successful discharge of her duties she needs more than sympathy and devotion, essential as these qualities are. Apprenticeship experience alone will not suffice. There must be both education and training in hospital, dispensary and field. Widening opportunities are making larger demands, changes in organization and methods of education are taking place, new schools are being created. Countries in which this type of training has not been developed are adopting modern ideas of teaching and of practical apprenticeship.

The debate of Beard versus Mayo, though it took place nearly four decades ago, is of more than mere historical interest. The fact that two such influential men engaged so spiritedly in the discussion of nursing education helped to focus attention on the needs of the profession and, no doubt, to formulate the attitudes of the profession itself. If Dr. Beard and Dr. Mayo were alive today they would look with the greatest interest at the new programs of our experimental age: the two-year curriculum now being offered, in many places, to certain qualified applicants; the courses in practical nursing with which Minnesota's school has pioneered; and the several advanced programs for preparation in the specialties of teaching and administration which Minnesota has also developed. Each would see that a growing profession must examine the ideas of all conscientious critics and put their good principles to work. And perhaps, as they parted, Dr. Beard and Dr. Mayo would glance at each other with smiles of mutual indulgence and say with one voice: "You see! I was right all the time."

6

Hercules among the Maidens

A PARTNERSHIP that had lasted for a dozen years was broken when Miss Powell left Minnesota, but Marion Vannier, who became successor to the senior member, was well equipped to carry on the tradition of the school and to maintain its atmosphere of warm encouragement to youthful effort. "I doubt," Alma Haupt once said, "if many schools ever had a team so close to its student body, so loved and so respected."

Miss Vannier's successor, in turn, proved to a director of the same kind — teacher, counselor, and source of bracing stimulation all in one. The values of sensitive consideration for students, loyalty to faculty, deep concern for academic standards, and sense of responsibility toward the future of the profession — these were Katharine Densford's values as well. To expand Alma Haupt's comment: there can be few schools whose records show so uninterrupted a pattern of harmonious personal relationships in the midst of strenuous enterprise or so good a temper in the midst of challenging problems.

The administration of Miss Vannier lasted for six years. Its concerns were ones that had long since become familiar. It must, first of all, demonstrate that a superior kind of training for the nurse pays dividends in service to the public. Second, it must urge faculty members to improve their qualifications and in doing so broaden opportunities for students. Third, it must improve the student body itself by making a conscious effort to attract the best kind of human material.

An answer to the first challenge came early in Miss Vannier's regime and it came in a form also familiar — that of near disaster.

74

During the summer and fall of 1924 and again in the winter of 1925 the Minneapolis community learned in a tragic way how great a need there was for awareness of the principles of health protection. An epidemic of virulent hemorrhagic smallpox swept across Minnesota, engulfing Minneapolis along with many other communities of the state. Eighteen cities scattered across the continent were also affected. Long continued neglect of the safeguard offered by vaccination was being bitterly punished.

Since 1883 Minnesota had had a law with many words but few teeth in it, which urged that "every person being the parent or guardian of any minor shall to the extent of any means that could properly be used cause such minor to be promptly, frequently and effectively vaccinated." Even this mild admonition had suffered a kind of progressive dedentition. It was regarded with such distaste by cranks that, in 1903, the state legislature had approved an "act to prevent compulsory vaccination and to prevent vaccination being made a condition precedent to school attendance." Tables of the Health Department show that the incidence of smallpox began soon thereafter to increase and in 1920 Minneapolis experienced an epidemic of mild type. Cases were many but illness was of short duration and the general public did not become sufficiently frightened to ask for protection. So, as an article in *Modern Medicine* has pointed out, "a fertile field for the virulent epidemic of 1924–25 was cultivated."

Every aspect of this outbreak was designed to breed panic. The epidemic proved to be atypical in several ways. Cases appeared out of backgrounds that would have been thought to be immaculate, among persons who had no idea that they had been exposed. The pattern of the illness was marked by violent symptoms leading to death in a hemorrhagic crisis. In such violent cases death came often within twenty-four hours, sometimes within twelve.

The Board of Health promptly began a vigorous campaign to reach unvaccinated citizens. Doctors and nurses worked all day and far into the night. They could "smell the smallpox cases as they came to the doors" of the Health Department and they "carried the odor in their memories" for the rest of their lives. With the cooperation of the Salvation Army, the city missions — and with the support of the newspapers which gave liberally of their space to forward the campaign — the "idea of vaccination was put across."

But the great burden of the disaster fell on the hospitals. Of the 1,500 cases in the city of Minneapolis 562 made their way to the Minneapolis General where the nurses of the university assumed by far the greatest share of responsibility for care. It was to be expected that these young women would accept the discipline of their profession and respond to its challenge. As Miss Vannier wrote in her annual report to the president, they handled the task of caring not merely for the smallpox victims but for all other infectious diseases admitted during the period "in a fine spirit of unselfish service." Not one "showed the slightest unwillingness to accept the depressing and difficult duty."

But the significant thing about their performance was its effectiveness. The "intelligent and sympathetic care" which as Miss Vannier testified, they had been able to offer kept the mortality rate from being as appalling as it might otherwise have been. *Journal-Lancet* reported that the number of deaths in Minneapolis had not been "alarmingly high." *Modern Medicine*, in a later investigation, found that "four-fifths of all deaths from smallpox in the local epidemic of 1924–25 were in those never vaccinated."

It is a tragic irony that one of the few victims who died violently despite the fact that she had been vaccinated was a student nurse from the university.

Nevertheless, the significance of the story is that care of the kind that only people with a superior kind of training can give had saved the community from the worst effects of the disaster. The case for high standards had been presented dramatically once more.

In March, 1925, when the smallpox epidemic was under control and the situation in the School of Nursing was as nearly placid as it was ever likely to be, Miss Vannier tried to resign. She may well have been prompted in part by the belief that a school on the university level should have a director who held a baccalaureate degree. Miss Vannier had not followed Miss Powell's example by returning frequently to school as student. But her success as administrator had been so great, particularly at the time of organization of the Central School, that no one was willing to see her go. The response to her resignation was one of complete dismay, and within a week she had agreed, under certain conditions, to withdraw it.

These conditions had chiefly to do with academic matters. She wanted "the continuance and support of the Central School." She desired that Dr. Beard, who was about to retire from the medical faculty, should somehow be continued as the school's guide even if it were necessary to create a title for him as "advisory member of the committee" on which he had worked so long. Problems with regard to Miss Vannier's hypersensitiveness were resolved by votes of confidence and the affairs of the school went on without interruption.

The appropriate effect of the director's conviction about the importance of degrees was that she urged the members of her staff to earn them and supported their efforts to do so. With Miss Vannier's help a group of Minnesota women were able so greatly to broaden their qualifications that they were later drawn into important work for the profession, either as directors of educational programs or as investigators of research problems.

A representative of this group was Barbara Thompson who had been involved in the school's history almost from its beginning. She had entered as a student in 1910 and been presented to the president as a graduate of its second class in 1913. Thereafter her development followed a pattern that became classic for Minnesotans. She served with the university base hospital in France and later with Evacuation Hospital, Unit 7. Back from the war, she joined Miss Vannier in helping to create the nursing service of Miller Hospital. The organization of the Central School brought her back into the university community where she served for many years as superintendent of nurses in the General Hospital.

Barbara Thompson followed the classic pattern also in her obsession with study. Perhaps the only boast that Miss Powell ever made was that she had earned her B.S. degree when she was fifty-one years old. Miss Thompson did not wait so long but took her baccalaureate degree at Minnesota in 1932. Meanwhile she found time to collaborate with Miss Vannier on a *Manual of Nursing Procedures.*

For more than twenty years Barbara Thompson helped to develop the educational program of her own university. Then, as a recognized leader, she was drawn away to posts of responsibility such as Minnesota could not, at the moment, offer her. She became first director of the Bureau of Educational Nursing, under the State Board of Health at Madison, Wisconsin, and later one of the several secretaries of the National League of Nursing Education. Later still, as Mrs. Sharpless, she continued, in her own vigorous substitute for retirement, to interest herself in nursing organizations and nursing problems.

The atmosphere of the "learning situation," within the School of Nursing became congenial, not to say positively seductive. Those who were closest to Miss Vannier became most deeply infected with the desire to explore new possibilities. Such a person was H. Phoebe Gordon who entered the school first as Miss Vannier's secretary and later became, in an important field, one of its major contributors.

Miss Gordon was a graduate of Wellesley College and her excellent academic background had filled her mind with interests which the duties of a secretary could not entirely satisfy. The arrival at Minnesota of Miss Vannier's successor, Katharine Densford, resulted in Miss Gordon's undertaking graduate study in psychometrics while she continued to do her full-time job in the school. To have a faculty of high personal achievement was one of the director's particular points of professional pride and Miss Densford constantly urged her associates to seek higher degrees.

It was a lively time in the university when Miss Gordon began to work for her master's degree under the direction of Professor Donald Paterson. During the late 1920's and early 1930's, the University of Minnesota stepped into leadership for the entire country in the scientific measurement of college aptitude. Dean John Black Johnston of the arts college turned the penetrating gaze of his chill blue eyes into all the dark corners where academic procedures had settled into unimaginative routine. He was determined to seek out an educational elite no matter how perversely the lights of superior students might be hidden under firmly planted bushels. Professor Paterson had been the dean's ally in creating psychological tests to be used in all aspects of student guidance. In this atmosphere of concern for investigation Miss Gordon worked until 1933 when she earned her master's degree in psychometrics.

In 1936 she accepted the position of assistant director of the Nursing Testing Division of the Psychological Corporation in New York. During the same period Miss Densford had been intent upon developing in the School of Nursing the principles and techniques of personnel service to students. To this comparatively new field Miss Gordon returned as student counselor in the school. Miss Densford and she collaborated so well in this task that they became coauthors — along with

E. G. Williamson, Minnesota's dean of students — of an important book: *Counseling in Schools of Nursing*. It is believed that Miss Gordon has the distinction of having been the first qualified, full-time counselor in a school of nursing.

Another addition to the faculty of the school in Miss Vannier's time was Deborah MacLurg (later Mrs. Julius Jensen). One of her contributions was to introduce into instruction at Minnesota the use of the case method. Adapted from the fundamental principle developed long before at Harvard for preparing the law student, the case method was then an innovation in the field of nursing. Coming to much fuller development in subsequent years, this particular tool for the solution of problems has great usefulness, as one contemporary expert has said, in helping "to develop the habit of analysis." The nurse student is confronted with an actual situation in the care of Patient A. She reviews all the materials involved in a perplexing crisis and explores alternative courses of action. In a group of students the suggestions of one are tested against the experience of others. Emphasis is placed on the facts of the crisis and the task is to find a solution exactly as the nurse would have to do on the job. The case method introduces the nurse student to that moment of decision when an active practitioner must draw quickly on all her knowledge of human relations and other skills in order to serve her patient well.

A third important figure in the dramatis personae of the nursing world who made her debut at Minnesota during Miss Vannier's administration of the school was Eula Butzerin. She arrived in 1924 straight from Teachers College, Columbia, to succeed Mrs. Mariette in responsibility for the public health nursing courses. This continued to be her task for thirteen years before she was invited to go first to the University of Chicago and later into the work of the nursing service of the national Red Cross in Washington. During that time she helped to develop a distinguished program and also to create an image of herself as a stimulating teacher that has endured ever since. Mary Beard of the Rockefeller Foundation once offered Miss Butzerin's accomplishment this unreserved endorsement:

I have heard it said often and I believe it to be true that the course in public health nursing given at the University of Minnesota fits a nurse for rural nursing better than any other. When a school has such a reputation as this, one nearly always finds that some one person connected with it has unusual qualities of leadership. Such a leader is Eula Butzerin. I should like to pay personal tribute to her and to the admirable course which she directs. Thoroughly grounded in principles and practice, this course has consistently grown with the changing needs of the public health field.

As a result of its readiness steadily to reappraise and improve its techniques, the School of Nursing earned praise from impartial observers. In 1926 Professor Abbie Turner of the department of physiology at Mount Holyoke spent ten days in regular attendance at classes and reported to the Rockefeller Foundation, as a member of its committee on nursing education, that the work done at Minnesota in the clinical teaching of medical nursing easily won first place among all schools. In the following year Mary Beard, also reporting to the Rockefeller Foundation, gave the school equally high marks.

The third major concern of Miss Vannier's regime — the ever-recurrent one of enrolling able students — was perhaps the most complicated of all. Many university minds concentrated on it and these minds were by no means in complete agreement about the issues or even about the first steps that might be taken toward solution of the fundamental question of what constituted promising material.

One of these minds belonged to Dean Lyon. He was a man who had lived all his life in the atmosphere of dedication to scholarship. He loved the well-ventilated, well-lighted place in which the scholar lives. So complete was this preoccupation with the interests of investigation that even his small summer cottage on the St. Croix River was likely to be transformed, over a weekend, into a seminar for consideration of the problems of education. Twelve or fourteen guests, assembled at random — scientists, writers, nonacademic neighbors, children and grandchildren — were likely to be drawn into discussions of the fundamental problems of human society.

It was to be expected that when Dean Lyon turned his attention to matters of nursing education he would have many original, and some disturbing, things to say.

When he had come to Minnesota as dean, the School of Nursing had been in existence for four years and Dr. Beard had been, during all that time, its close adviser. Indeed, he seemed always to be well within earshot of the slightest whisper of difficulty and he appeared to offer counsel as quickly as the desire for it had been formed. Dean Lyon regarded this faithful colleague as a specialist in the field of nursing and delegated to him responsibility for such matters.

This did not mean, however, that Dean Lyon lacked interest. Even before the establishment of the school at Minnesota he had been preaching the doctrine of the importance of nursing education wherever he could find an audience. He had accepted innumerable calls to serve on committees, both those that were local to Minnesota and those that operated on a national level. As he once said: "I have studied nursing education, read about it and talked about it with many people. Like the hero of Greek legend — was it Hercules? — I have gone about in female attire, figuratively speaking — spinning with the maidens."

This intimate exposure to the subject steadily deepened his conviction that what the profession needed to do was to throw out a dragnet and capture the most promising kind of prospective nurses wherever these could be found. His concern with quality was no greater, but also no less in the selection of nursing students than it was in the selection of men to be trained in medicine. To the end of his career he continued to look for a better basis than any yet found for admission to medical schools. In what he called his "swan song," an address delivered before the Congress on Medical Education in 1936, he said: "Until we are surer of our raw material, more exacting in our inspection of it, more clear about what our product should be, the medical profession will average lower than it should in the great field test that goes on today in the fight for better health."

Dean Lyon was not convinced that existing standards for entrance to schools of nursing were the right ones by which to judge qualification. As his fellow dean, Dr. W. C. Rappleye, of the College of Physicians and Surgeons at Columbia University, had pointed out: "The remarkable increase in medical knowledge during recent years has added greatly to what a nurse is expected to know and to what she is expected to do." Lyon began to wonder if a type of student more mature than the average high school graduate could claim to be might not serve present-day needs better. He made so bold as to say so in a letter to Dr. Beard. He wrote:

This country needs nurses. We need pupils in our school. No one wants poorly trained nurses or ones lacking in intelligence. The question is whether we are getting as intelligent and as properly trained nurses as possible. This raises the question as to how intelligence and proper preparation may be tested.

Quite certainly, he believed, a high school diploma represented no badge of distinction. "On the whole graduates of high school are not a highly selective group. This is shown by the large percentage of failures in the junior colleges." Similarly it seemed clear to the dean that some people without high school diplomas had "both ability and preparation" to which their "accomplishments in life" attested. The School of Nursing "should be particularly careful not to close the door of opportunity against this class of able students."

What he wanted to see was a greater flexibility in selection. Besides high school graduates, two other groups should be considered; those who were able to pass a special entrance examination and "women at least twenty-one years old who take a psychologic test and are recommended by the psychology department." He would have had them take also an examination in English composition, success in which would admit them to the school as "unclassed students." After two quarters they might then be (a) accepted as regular students (b) be required to prolong the period of training or (c) be rejected.

These experimental ideas were in complete sympathy with the principles which Dean Johnston was in the process of developing in the arts college. Each of these men had in his temperament so little of the intellectual snob that devoted followers of the principles of the guild found them difficult to understand. But the objective of Dean Johnston and Dean Lyon was, quite simply, to get the best wherever the best could be found.

All this talk worried Dr. Beard who remembered the controversy with Dr. Mayo and feared that another subversive move toward lowering standards threatened. He did not want to see doubtful experiments made anywhere. But if the deans must engage in occult rites, let them — he said bluntly — not make the School of Nursing their "sacrificial goat."

He need not have worried. Dean Johnston's tests, soon to become famous and influential the country over, were intended to push standards up, not down. They examined candidates, as individuals, and appraised their demonstrated aptitudes without being content to accept so doubtful a witness to competence as Dean Johnston believed a high school diploma to be.

The debate between Dean Lyon and Dr. Beard had the stimulating effect of inviting many educators to begin to entertain experimental ideas for the future like that of training practical nurses in a university school. But it did not change basic regulations. The bulletin of the School of Nursing continued to announce that "the presentation of a high school diploma" was a prerequisite for the consideration of a candidate. Just a little reticently it mentioned the possibility of admission by special examination, saying that further information could be obtained by request.

The years of Miss Vannier's administration were ones of steady development within a pattern already established. The level of faculty achievement rose. The curriculum was kept up to date; opportunities were broadened. In 1928, Barbara Thompson, acting director during Miss Vannier's sabbatical leave, announced an innovation. For the first time the School of Nursing offered regular courses in summer school. These were Administration in Schools of Nursing and Ward Teaching and Administration. In the academic year 1929–30, the five-year (eighteen-quarter) course was completely revised by a committee made up of Dean Lyon, Dean Melvin Haggerty of the College of Education, Dr. Diehl, Miss Butzerin, and Miss Vannier.

But while concern for the nurse's professional well-being broadened, concern for physical welfare was at a standstill. The university owned land on which to build a new residence; it had even gone so far as to ask architects to draw up plans. But at each successive session of the legislature the request for funds with which to make a start was relegated to the bottom of the list of university requirements — and ignored. A stoical but nonetheless plaintive theme runs through Miss Vannier's reports. Housing the nurses in scattered units — there were thirteen of them now — created baffling problems of administration. The students continued to endure physical hardships of a kind associated in most people's imaginations only with log cabins on lonely frontiers.

And still the miserable conditions continued to prevail.

A student with an ironic turn of mind listed for *Alumnae Quarterly* in April, 1929, the joys of living in one of the homes: refreshing breezes that blew through the livingroom out of the fireplace; pipes that provided inexpensive diversions by freezing and bursting at opportune moments; other pipes that made harmonious music all night long; water that dripped constantly from the ceiling providing showerbaths for those who were just in the process of washing out their stockings. There were such other exhilarating circumstances as standing in the cold at 2:45 in the morning en route to meet an emergency in the operating room, while heavy truck traffic on Washington Avenue refused to give way and allow a nurse to cross the street.

The bulletin of the School of Nursing for the summer session of 1930 listed among its courses two of chief importance, Organization and Administration, to be taught by Katharine J. Densford, assistant dean and associate director of the Nursing Service of Cook County Hospital, Chicago; and Teaching and Supervising in Schools of Nursing, to be taught by Lucile Petry, instructor in the School of Nursing.

These announcements actually foretold much about the shape of things to come. During the next three decades the names of Miss Densford and Miss Petry were to be conspicuously associated with the development of nursing education. Though the announcement was yet to be made, Miss Densford had already been chosen as Miss Vannier's successor. Miss Petry had been in residence just a year as faculty member.

The date, July 1, 1930, is a convenient one to set between two distinct phases in the progress of the School of Nursing. In its twenty-first year it had indeed "reached its majority" and was ready, under new leadership, to assume the responsibilities of a quite new era in its history.

7

Portrait of a Giver

❧ IN A LETTER to his mother, the novelist Thomas Wolfe once divided the human race into large categories, the givers and the takers.

Though the definition, "one who is oriented toward service," might seem to some a more adequate identification of a member of the first group, there are advantages to the novelist's word. The chief of these is that it stresses the spontaneity with which the true giver gives — the ungrudging readiness of his identification with others.

Katharine Densford would seem to have been oriented toward service almost from the moment of her birth. On her father's moderately large farm near the town of Crothersville, Indiana, she had a good life. In its generous milieu she enjoyed the advantages of being a "much loved, much wanted" child, of having responsibility and independence entrusted to her in the same neat package of family attitudes, and of living comfortably, though she assumed the farm way of life to be less affluent than actually it was. Her own education began in a day when parents sent their children to school if it was entirely convenient to do so, not because an appointed hour had been reached. Once she interrupted a highly promising academic career to go home, in a family emergency, to become her father's housekeeper. Both father and elder brother unhesitatingly surrendered their checkbooks and left to a girl in her early teens all decisions concerned with the family budget.

Out of a training in which elements that were gracious blended so easily with ones that were exacting, there developed in the young woman's mind a personal philosophy well suited to one who was to become an educator. To Katharine Densford it seemed clear, as she examined her own experience, that most human beings are well-intentioned; that differences of education and opportunity produce differences in thought and behavior; that this variety is to be encouraged, rather than deplored, not merely for its piquancy but for the richness that it adds to human life; that the chance to serve any group in society should be regarded as a benefit conferred, not a burden inflicted; and that to travel hopefully in the light of the race's wisdom toward a foreseen objective may be said to be the purpose of living.

It was in the serenely happy home of her parents that Katharine Densford began to develop this philosophy. Her mother was the descendant of a long line of professional people — lawyers, ministers, engineers, government officials, and teachers. She herself was a fine musician, an active leader in community affairs, a tireless learner who, when she was not occupied otherwise with the duties of a household manager, always "had a book in her hands." The loss of this mother was an early sorrow, but the responsibility of succeeding her in the service of a devoted, busy father was for Katharine Densford a privilege in which to take pride.

An intimate friend of her mother became Katharine Densford's first important educational mentor. Catherine Cox (Kochenour) was dean of Oxford College for Women, across the Indiana-Ohio border, which included a preparatory department, and it was under her guidance that Katharine Densford was led into unusual opportunities to demonstrate the sincerity of her own philosophy of service. When Miss Cox was persuaded to become dean of a girls' "industrial school" it was to this aptest of her pupils that she turned in her first emergency. The name of this institution resulted from a semantic triumph over grim realities, for this was actually a home for delinquents. Among the victims of social inequality to be found in it were children as young as eight, and Miss Densford was asked to become teacher of its fourth, fifth, and sixth grades. She was instructor also in what was then called manual training.

The particular reason for the sudden call was that Miss Densford's predecessor had been vigorously kicked and then threatened with a butcher knife by a particularly resolute member of the sixth grade. The teacher had retreated abruptly to a world less charged with frustrated passion.

Into this atmosphere — one from which Dickens might have drawn another scene for *Oliver Twist* or *Nicholas Nickleby* — Miss Densford went armed with an indestructible belief in the inherent goodness of the

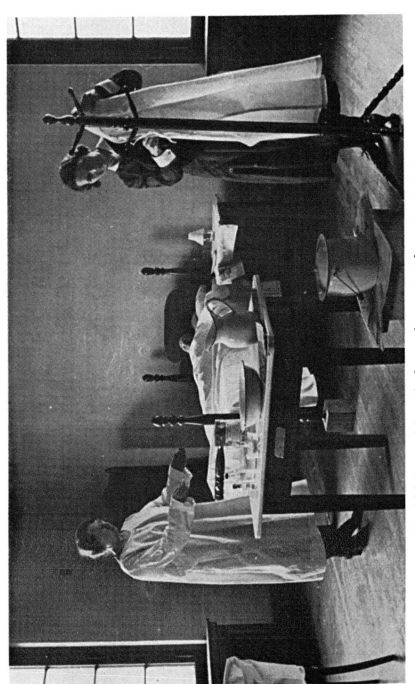

Pearl McIver and Sena Anderson demonstrate home treatment of communicable disease

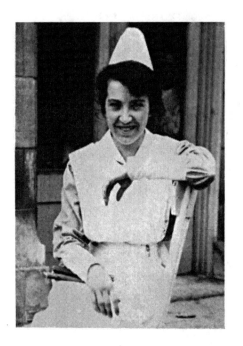

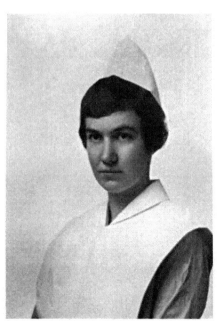

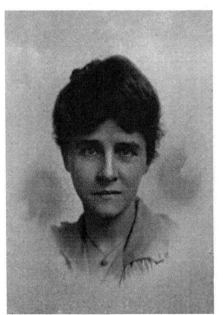

Top left, Alma Haupt, class of 1919, pioneer teacher in the School of Nursing. *Top right*, Anna Jones Mariette, class of 1919. *Bottom*, Dorothy Slade Kurtzman, creator of the University's first course in public health

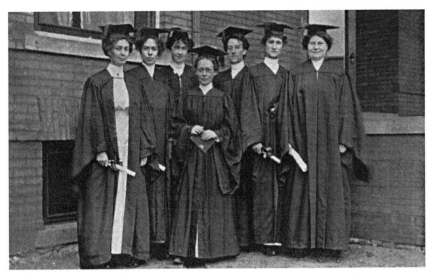

The class of 1912: Olga Belta Skonnard, Mary E. Mark, Elizabeth Burns, (Miss Powell), Lena Belle Stewart, Carolyn Schwarg, Margaret Ames

Elliot Hospital in the early twenties

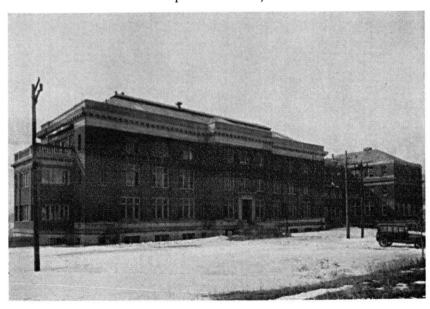

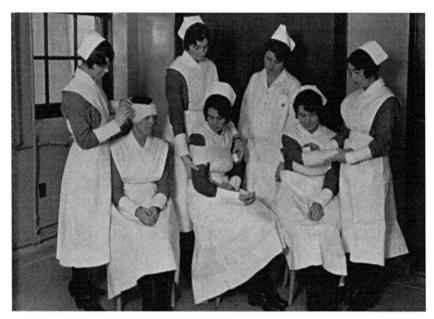

Student nurses of the early thirties demonstrate bandaging techniques

Nurses' prize-winning float in the 1933 Homecoming parade

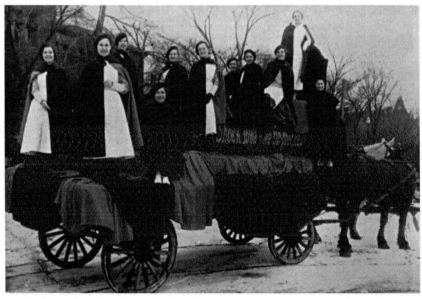

individual human being. She felt the need of no other weapon even against butcher knives. And, indeed, for her, this conviction worked. Her pupils became her friends. Even when some "hard cases" had to be removed to the women's prison they did not cease to have her interest and good will. It was, at the time, her favorite joke that she had more friends in prison than anywhere else.

What she plucked out of this experience was further assurance that human beings respond to liking and to trust. With modest gratification, she saw a high proportion of these pupils rehabilitated by the care they received, not only from herself and other teachers like her, but from the administrator and from the field supervisor of the school. Many of these girls went into adoptive homes, or into jobs, and became useful citizens. They had been taught, by consideration, to slough off and discard the ill effects of sordid upbringing. At no time had the atmosphere of the home for delinquent girls seemed depressing. To Katharine Densford this first in a long succession of classrooms was one in which all the hopeful convictions of an educator-in-the-making found bright reward and justification.

At the end of two years, however, her father and brother decided that this could not go on. Education had its own proper claim upon a candidate who had already shown an aptitude for honors. Oxford College for Women had placed emphasis on languages and Katharine Densford had done particularly well in Latin, Greek, and German. Her Latin teacher, a fearsome disciplinarian, had a curious system of marking which set a certain number of correct answers as the perfect score and allowed bonus credit for more correct answers than the required number. Miss Densford often received 120 in Latin. It did no good for the president to protest that there was — there could be — no such mark. This stubborn descendant of all the Prussians, in residence at Oxford College, continued to record for her best pupil pluperfect grades in Latin. To such a student the advantages of formal training must not be denied — so the Densford men decided.

This group solidarity again had the effect of nourishing in a sensitive young woman a sense of the interdependence of human beings. Even casual outsiders tended to notice with pleasure the mutual confidence of brother and sister. Once when Katharine Densford was at home on vacation her brother went with her to a store in Indianapolis to buy a suit. It must be, she had decided, of good stuff and cost only what a strict budget allowed. The first condition was met by an attractive item, but not the second. Miss Densford refused to buy the otherwise ideal suit the price of which she considered to be beyond her means. "Get it," her brother kept urging, "I'll pay the difference."

The owner of the store, happening to overhear part of this interchange, assumed it to be a colloquy between devoted husband and wife. When he learned that these were brother and sister he was suddenly inspired to say "Let *me* pay the difference." Anyone who had earned such loyalty from a mere brother should, the merchant insisted, have what she wanted.

The story has a significance to match its charm. For the willingness to "pay the difference" for a fellow creature in need may well be considered to be the basis of social responsibility.

At Miami University Katharine Densford briskly finished three years' work in two and felt that she had had her share of academic training. But her father insisted that she was entitled to another year of preparation. So she went to the University of Chicago and earned a master's degree in a favorite subject, history.

As Katharine Densford saw her world, it was a charmed path that she walked thereafter. "The eye sees what it brings with it the power to see" and, in the Michigan town of the Upper Peninsula where she went to teach Latin and German in the high school, there were many "delightful experiences." The people, still close to the pioneer way of life, seemed to be no rubber stamps of conformity in matters of taste or judgment. Fresh, forthright, self-reliant, and humorous, they made up a constantly surprising American tradition as they went along. Katharine Densford enjoyed it all as participant in a drama that was good because it contained the elements — harsh as well as pleasant — that make up the sum of human life.

But the teaching of history also had its attractions and it was to seize an opportunity to do so that Katharine Densford went, for two years, to Bismarck, North Dakota.

There the events of 1917 swept disruptingly across her quiet path as they swept along every highroad and byroad of America. Surprised out of its provincialism, the United States went to war and a conscientious, vigorously healthy young woman could see for herself no possibility but that of going, too.

Again it was a sense of social solidarity that made the decision spring spontaneously out of the inevitable. Katharine Densford's father was ready to serve on the farm under command of the slogan, Food Will Win the War. Her brother and sister were also committed to civilian responsibilities. Only she could put on the uniform. She chose the one that the emergency urged upon women, that of a nurse in training.

She went to the Vassar Training Camp which was open only to college graduates. This feature of the plan set up by Miss Nutting's committee, under the council for National Defense, was designed to lure American women of superior training to a neglected field. But, once it got them the program showed no inclination to coddle them. The routine was rigorous. At 6:00 in the morning four hundred young women were bugled shrilly out of bed. At 6:15 they had aired their rooms; at 6:30 they had been through setting-up exercises that discovered nerves and sinews previously unused by women who had spent their adolescence bent over nothing more demanding than books; by 7:00 they had showered and breakfasted; by 7:30 they had dusted everything in sight and reach so that Poughkeepsie shone as never before in all its history. They were then ready for the day's work which continued for fifteen hours.

When the Fourth of July arrived, the commanding officer of the Vassar Training Camp (Dean Mills, borrowed from the headship of the department of social sciences) offered candidates a choice as to whether they would take a holiday or go on with the regular program. From the depths of four hundred weary bodies there issued a groan in unison, but four hundred hands went up in a vote for patriotic duty. They kept no holiday at Vassar.

In the midst of this experience Katharine Densford realized that patriotic duty had in fact led her into a way of life that seemed more rewarding than any other could be. Its very rigors spoke eloquently of humanity's great need of care. When she went to the University of Cincinnati School (later College) of Nursing and Health to continue her training under the war plan she knew that she must be a nurse for the rest of her days.

There she had the first of a series of associations with a woman who belonged to the long line of women whom Canada has contributed to the development of nursing education. Laura Logan, who was to become, after Adelaide Nutting, the second professor of nursing in a university, seemed to feel that a kind of apostolic responsibility had descended to her straight from Florence Nightingale. From doctors she evoked not merely respect but a kind of awe. One such, himself a scrupulous and demanding man of science, once said of her, when she first blazed into his ken as director of a new job, that in six months she had made the whole place over, sweeping out all the cobwebs of lassitude and conformity.

It was inevitable that a man of imagination should have been impressed, for Miss Logan was in every respect ahead of her time. Into her program she introduced courses in communicable disease nursing, in psychiatric nursing, in public health nursing, and in physical and occupational therapy at a time when such refinements of instruction were undreamed of in most schools and a quarter of a century was to pass before they became features of the average curriculum.

It was Miss Logan's belief that a hospital which ministered to the poor offered a training center par excellence because it opened experience on the whole range of human enterprise in the battle with disease. It must conserve, more jealously than any other institution, the best nursing tradition and maintain its facilities at the highest point of efficiency. At Cincinnati Miss Logan created many a model for others to imitate.

From her work as student nurse Katharine Densford moved directly into a position of directive responsibility as head nurse and then out into the general field of public health nursing. Under the Red Cross she covered one third of an Ohio county, carrying into obscure corners the news of facilities offered by public health branches of its service.

The American tradition of self-reliance had allowed the concept of social service to be slow in developing in the rural districts. But the frightening memory of the flu epidemic had changed all that. Now everything had to be done in a tremendous hurry in order to forestall another such disaster. Trained workers were few and upon them rested the heavy responsibility of indoctrinating the whole citizenry in the principles of a benevolent revolution. Doctors had to be persuaded to respect these efforts. Mothers had to be urged into clinics to learn the fundamentals of infant welfare, even the rudimentary ones of preparing adequate meals. Undernourishment was a daily problem even in communities that seemed self-respecting and orderly.

From many quarters response came gratefully. On one occasion Katharine Densford went on a routine visit to a home where she found that disaster had struck from all sides simultaneously. A pregnant mother was proving herself to be entirely inadequate to the care of a husband, suffering, as she failed to understand, from pneumonia and a child dangerously ill from malnutrition. Quick action was required of a kind which a nurse is not, in ordinary circumstances, authorized to take. Katharine Densford, alert to immediate danger and fully aware of what must be done, called the neighborhood doctor on the telephone and found him glad to delegate to her responsibility for giving treatment.

This work seemed so important to Katharine Densford that she was reluctant to leave it. Several times she refused offers of teaching jobs because she enjoyed active association with people who were pitifully uninstructed but eager to learn. However, the field of the missionary is a specialized one. Other assignments seemed to touch upon all its values and at the same time to offer a broader opportunity for service. She took such a job.

It was in a tuberculosis sanatorium and an incidental result of her taking up this new work was that Katharine Densford became a frequent contributor of magazine articles to the literature of the field.

But in the daily work of the sanatorium she encountered curious resistance. No one had wanted her in this institution, she had simply been sent. As an active threat to the status quo she was resented and the attendants, who regarded themselves as being in possession, set their faces grimly against innovations that might down-grade their own prestige.

On her first day at work a red-haired goddess descended out of her X-ray machine in a nearby department and demanded one of the three chairs which furnished Miss Densford's office. It was a gesture intended vaguely at sabotage but the newcomer at the sanatorium only said mildly, "I can get on without them." Disarmed of her Irish aggressiveness the enemy soon became an ally who helped to spread the gospel of the new dispensation.

Miss Densford had need of an ally. She had need also of those talents as diplomatist which her private philosophy had given her. The sanatorium had little in the way of trained personnel. Attendants performed the functions of head nurses. As student nurses were brought in, their way had to be smoothed for them. Placatingly, Miss Densford pointed out that this was a cooperative project. Each group had something to give the other. The attendants knew the patients and had many insights

91

into their psychological needs. The students were in command of new techniques that could also be useful. A kind of benevolent erosion gradually wore resistance away. When, a little at a time, trained people replaced attendants as head nurses even this was not resented.

It was almost inevitable that Miss Densford should eventually rejoin Miss Logan. When the latter became head of the Illinois Training School for Nurses (later the Cook County School of Nursing) she called Katharine Densford to the post of assistant dean and associate director.

There, too, the feeling of the guild was strong. As the oldest institution of its kind west of the Alleghenies, the Illinois School was jealous of its prestige. "Are you a graduate of the I.T.S.?" was a challenge flung so often at Katharine Densford's head that she became an artist at dodging what were meant to be slurs. To dare to become a teacher at Illinois without first having been a student there was incredible pretension. Waiting for an opportune moment to take a stand she met the question still once more. This time she stopped firmly in her tracks and answered with deliberate defiance, "No, I'm not. I'm sorry." "Well," said the other nurse whom Miss Densford knew to be an Illinois graduate, "I'm not sorry. We need new blood around here."

They got it and they got the innovations as well. But for these not all the students were equally grateful.

At Illinois there never had been a course of any kind in community nursing. Laura Logan and the faculty, feeling this to be a serious gap in the students' training, created one. On the first day when the class was to meet the instructor, Miss Densford walked through a lounge on the way to the appointed place and found all of the young nurses assembled there.

"We are meeting in room so-and-so," she said cheerfully.

No one moved.

Feeling as though she had somehow momentarily lost contact with reality she tried again.

"Shall we go in now?" she said and made a movement as though to lead the way.

Then someone was nudged forward to act as spokesman. "We aren't going in," this young woman said. "Your course wasn't part of the curriculum when we enrolled and we don't have to take it."

A cloud of apprehension descended upon Miss Densford as she realized that she had a strike on her hands. All the effort of the faculty had been misinterpreted; what had been offered to the students as an opportunity had been received as a burden, almost as an imposition.

Once more the sacredness of the status quo was at stake. What had been done in the past must be done in the future. Like so many stern-lipped Cordelias, the student nurses loved their tradition, their profession, and their school "according to its desert — no more, no less." They did not rise to follow.

It is an awkward moment of decision. Katharine Densford, acting under the discipline of a long-cultivated faith in human nature, chose to renounce authority in favor of tact. As she once described her situation, more graphically, she "scrambled for base."

"Well," she suggested, "shall we just go in for the first class and then talk it over?"

By invoking the principle of fair play in which she herself had always believed profoundly, she gained a kind of armistice. A group of unpersuaded, but undefiant students followed her into the classroom.

An hour later they left it — converts. What Katharine Densford had explained was that this was no punishment intended arbitrarily to increase the load of classwork. The hope was to offer a broader background. Public health nursing offered a field of new opportunity. Above all, the material of such a course was in itself interesting, dramatic, and intensely human. Her own enthusiasm and skillful presentation enabled her to make this felt as an immediate and rewarding justification of study.

There were no more strikes at the Illinois Training School though this was far from being the last extension of the training program.

For five years Miss Densford continued to work in this stimulating atmosphere. In the course of its strenuous routine she had wide experience in fields that were not strictly her own. Once in the unexpected absence of the bookkeeper she and another assistant to Miss Logan had to assume the responsibility of making up the institution's million-dollar payroll though neither had had previous training for the task. "We should charge you for this service," one of them said dryly to a member of the board of directors. Looking almost enviously at their statement in which she could find no mistake, the director answered: "We should charge *you* for this course in accounting."

It was indeed a unique course in institutional management, rich in detail, broad in scope which the Illinois Training School had to give a young woman who was always ready to catch up any opportunity for experience and for service.

One day in 1930 Miss Densford was invited with other faculty members to join Miss Logan and two guests at lunch. Men from Minnesota were visiting the school, she was told — Dean Lyon and Mr. Paul Fesler, administrator of the university hospitals.

What she did not know was that she was being observed by members of a committee looking for a new director of the university's School of Nursing. When the offer came Miss Densford accepted it as she had accepted every preceding call to service because that was what a responsible person did.

It was appropriate that the word of parting from one task and of salute to Katharine Densford at the beginning of another should be spoken of by her mentor of many years, Laura Logan. In the *Illinois State Nurses' Association Bulletin* Miss Logan wrote an appreciation of her associate in which she practiced, very adroitly, the "noble art of praise." The editorial speaks of Katharine Densford's student days as "filled with enthusiasm and prodigious accomplishment"; of her work in various agencies in the roles of teacher, organizer, and executive as having made "far reaching contributions"; of her service to the Education Committee of the National League of Nursing Education as showing "sound judgment and the qualities of leadership."

The effective final paragraph anticipated all the judgments that were presently to be made of Miss Densford at Minnesota. "The spirit and personality" of this young woman Miss Logan found difficult to describe but then proceeded to describe them aptly: "Her personal beauty, dignity, sweetness and loyalty," she said, "are of a rare quality. Like Marius, the Epicurean, she ever 'selects from the more select' in working out her life pattern and withal carrying more than her own end of the load."

8

Education versus Catastrophe

H. G. WELLS once described human history as being a race between education and catastrophe. The events of the 1930's were to prove that he was alarmingly right, and before the decade was over there had been much reason to fear that the prize might be lost to those who ran in the name of civilization. But even in the first years of the decade there were more than enough obstacles in the way of educators to make the outcome seem dubious. For the depression that followed the stock market crash of 1929 had cast its deep shadow over the outlook for the future, and in that darkness the rights of education were often obscured.

When she took up her work as director of the School of Nursing at Minnesota Katharine Densford had reason to know immediately that she was engaged in an endurance contest between positive and negative attitudes toward education. Throughout her whole career she faced problems of reduced budgets and shortages of staff. As war followed depression and sharp competition from other units of a university system constantly hedged her efforts round, she displayed inexhaustible resources of energy and persistence in making up the difference between the readily obtainable and the ideal. When she needed money that the university budget could not give, she got it from foundations, federal agencies, and friends. When she needed teachers whose salaries could not be paid out of funds that lay open to her, she added them to her faculty anyway and then explored outside means of supporting the expense.

She refused to believe that the depression had quite empty hands. There must be ways of coaxing effort out of its lethargy. Need could be balanced against need in the invention of previously untried procedures. More than once she demonstrated that, if it were deftly persuaded, the depression itself might show a golden hand.

Her first full statement of purpose, made to her dean shortly after her arrival in Minnesota, charted the direction she hoped to take toward three objectives: first, to maintain the standards already established; second, to build up a faculty of superior academic achievement; third, to reform curriculums in acknowledgement of the increased responsibilities of the nurse. All must be accomplished simultaneously. But emphasis must be put, at the start, on the problem of bringing together a group of teachers who had been prepared specifically for the work of teaching.

Though the faculty of early years had shown individual abilities of a high order, Miss Densford was disturbed by the fact that only eleven per cent of its members, in 1930, had preparation beyond that of the undergraduate course. A total of thirty per cent had had work on the university level or were taking classes in the extension division. This was a good showing for schools of the time but, for Miss Densford, it was far from being good enough.

What the director wanted was more teachers of the kind represented by her colleague, Lucile Petry (Leone). Together, these two believers in the value of higher education set out to find and to bring into the School of Nursing more women with their own kind of academic background.

Lucile Petry Leone, in the course of a career that has lasted three decades and is still in full swing, has earned many distinctions some of which are unique. She was the first woman to be appointed an assistant surgeon general of the United States Public Health Service; the first to have been chief of a division of the Public Health Service; the first — and so far, the only — person to be appointed to the post, created in 1945, of Chief Nurse Officer.

Twelve years of Mrs. Leone's professional life were spent at Minnesota. During that time she added tremendously to the prestige of the School of Nursing by helping to build up a solid and a broad program of instruction. Besides that invaluable contribution, she inducted so many students into the sorority of teaching leadership that their influence has been felt, quite literally, around the world.

The post of high distinction in the service of the United States which Mrs. Leone fills entitles her, in wartime and on ceremonial occasions, to wear the uniform either of a general in the army or an admiral in the navy. Yet there is nothing formidable about her unless it be her capacity for work. She is more at home in the civilian dress of a small, chic, pretty woman whose distinguishing characteristics are an enormous vitality; a voice which, to borrow Shakespeare's description, is "ever soft, gentle and low"; and a confiding manner which suggests that, to the resolute, any new effort is possible and every new effort is pleasurable.

The steps by which she became such a person presented themselves to Lucile Petry as ones that called only for spontaneous expressions of energy though each called, actually, for a display of unusual adaptability. In the home of her intellectually alert parents (her father was principal of a high school in a Delaware town) she lived in an atmosphere that encouraged lively interests of every kind. Among them were English literature, science, and any sort of part-time job that could use a pair of dextrous hands. She entered the University of Delaware in 1920 with no foregone conclusion about which of many attractions of the world's work she would want permanently — teaching philosophy, perhaps, or experimenting in scientific research.

But at the end of two years she had discovered that an ivory tower would be too unpeopled for her satisfaction; further it would have in it too little of the chaos that made daily life dramatic and worth trying to put in order. To her father's intense surprise she announced that she wanted to become a nurse. Here, she felt instinctually, was a work which engaged the intellect, the imagination, the heart, and the hands simultaneously. It *was* for her.

Her father continued to raise doubts. To quiet their echo in her own mind, she spent the summer after her sophomore year in college carrying trays, scrubbing the faces of old men who looked like Rembrandt drawings but whose actuality presented pungences less attractive, administering hypodermic injections without previous instruction (her aptitude for learning science "by the book" helped through this ordeal), making her own uniforms, earning twenty dollars a month, and becoming more sure, minute by minute, that she had found her vocation.

After earning her B.A. at Delaware she immediately entered the School of Nursing at Johns Hopkins (there was a period of just four days between the closing of one classroom door and the opening of another). Her record again was high and she went — one is tempted to say, romping — from scholarship to scholarship. After graduating from the training course, she received a grant to work for her M.A. at Teachers College, Columbia. The degree was hers in 1929 and, after spending a summer at Yale as assistant supervisor of clinical instruction in its school, she accepted Miss Vannier's invitation to come to Minnesota.

Her success as a teacher was immediately assured. A pupil of those earlier days retains a vivid image of her as she "paced up and down before her students, hands clasped behind her back," throwing off sparks of illumination seized from the minds of educators all the way from Plato to John Dewey and Bertrand Russell. In her course, Methods of Teaching, she followed no rigid, stereotyped routine but rather alerted the intelligences of those in her classroom by questioning them and by inviting their questions. She urged them to discover for themselves the significance of "the impact made by the flying age on the health problems of the universe." One of her important assets was "a great understanding of her students" by which she "helped them to see that nursing has content in itself." Its meaning cannot be appended, as footnote "to the outline of a medical lecture." Filled with ideas and overflowing with convictions, Lucile Petry's own philosophy of nursing was communicated to her students. A nurse, she said, quoting Harry Emerson Fosdick, nurses as much by what she *is* as by what she *does*. "We cannot separate in a nurse's experience those activities that make her a fine person from those which make her a fine nurse."

Miss Petry's own activities made her an enormously useful collaborator in all of the director's plans for improvement in the program of the school. A serious fault in the sequence of instruction which Miss Densford pointed out to her faculty was that, in traditional practice, a course in disease seldom coincided with a course in nursing. The result was that the student often had what Dean Lyon once described as "hazy and inadequate notions about the disease conditions" which it was her task to treat.

To close this gap between phases of theoretical and practical instruction Miss Densford and her faculty revised the basic curriculum in major ways so that, in each service, classwork either preceded or coincided with clinical experience. This correlation was made possible by a system of rotation through the services. Assignments to class and clinical experience were henceforth made for the entire three-year course at the beginning of each student's program. No longer was there the old vague and seemingly aimless leaping back and forth over the gap, a form of exercise too closely resembling that of jumping at conclusions. Method had bridged the difference.

It was Lucile Petry's preoccupation with the primary responsibility of patient care that prompted her to urge these changes. Like Katharine Densford she was determined that the rights of the sick man, woman, or child should never be lost to sight as supreme and that, in the ordering of hospital routine, the convenience of no other figure in the daily drama should be allowed to take precedence.

Miss Densford had received this gospel from her mentor, Laura Logan. That eminently sensible woman had never deviated from the principle. Once, when she was being interviewed by the Civil Service Commission for the position of director of the University of Cincinnati College of Nursing and Health, a shrewd man had thought to baffle her with the question: "Which do you consider more important — the patient or the student?" Miss Logan had answered promptly: "To neglect the student of today is to neglect the patient of tomorrow."

That the indivisibility of teaching and practice may not always be clear from special angles of vision, Miss Densford frequently reminded her colleagues. In an article, written for *Postgraduate Medicine* in 1954, she asked the question: Do We Take Each Other For Granted? She pointed out that, in a recent appraisal of its accomplishments, the Medical Association had "focused attention — and rightly so — on the doctor," but "slight, if any reference was made to other members of the health team — to chemists, to physicists, to nurses, to hospital administrators. Shortly after, a hospital association had held its annual meeting. One page of its program was devoted to a graphic portrayal of the hospital patient surrounded by the hospital personnel contributing to his welfare. Among them were hospital administrator, social worker, physical therapist, nutritionist and nurse — but not a sign of a physician." A short time later: "A large group of nurses, discussing the care of the patient and the many groups contributing to that care, also made a list. The group was sizeable. But here, too, no physician was on the list."

Warned by such examples of myopia, the School of Nursing at Minnesota has always undertaken to make it clear to students that the health team must function as a unit; that the nurse must always be aware of her role as a contributor to the work and as a member of the team.

But always the central figure of the drama is the woman waiting to deliver a child, the man in need of psychological rehabilitation after dismaying illness, the old man facing adjustment to the idea of permanent incapacitation, the young man needing care for a body broken in an accident, the young girl facing an operation, the child needing sympathy — in short, *the patient.*

This concept of "total care" — in contrast to care of routine adequacy — prompted important improvements in curriculums during the 1930's. Dean Lyon, among others, had pointed out the fact that too few women were being prepared for exacting jobs "in the various fields of specialized nursing endeavor." The list of such assignments included those of supervisors in medical nursing, surgical nursing, pediatric nursing, maternity nursing, and in the work of the operating room.

Here, again, the conditions of the depression threatened the rights of education. All institutions were crying poverty and suggestions with regard to new projects that might prove to be expensive were met by administrators with the blank look of incredulity. This, they insisted, was a time for curtailment, not for expansion.

But directors of schools of nursing were not to be easily turned away from the important objective of the profession which was "to develop nursing on a professional and collegiate level" farther than the efforts of the previous two decades had been able to do. Miss Densford, in particular, showed a patience — backed by imagination, resourcefulness and persistence — which managed to circumvent difficulties.

In the early years of the 1930's many graduate nurses could not find work. Though their services were needed more than ever before, in a time of adversity when psychosomatic illness greatly increased the usual number of the sick, an average man felt that he had no money with which to pay for care. Nurses swelled the ranks of the unemployed.

Educators saw an opportunity to put this enforced idleness to productive use. The University of Minnesota encouraged young people to return to school, supporting their studies, in part, with funds from the state government and, later, the federal government.

Through Miss Densford's enterprise similar opportunities were opened to professional nurses for postgraduate study in clinical areas. Ambitious young women were enabled to enter service in any of the hospitals associated with the university's programs. A bona fide student of the university in every sense, the nurse was assigned to thirty hours a week of clinical experience during the first ten months of her preparation and for forty-eight hours a week during a two-month period of administrative experience. In return for her contribution to the hospital she received board, room, and laundry service, plus an allowance of $10 a month. The university entered her on its rolls tuition-free. By successful completion of four quarters of work under this plan, the student earned between twenty and thirty academic credits. These could be applied toward a baccalaureate degree. The record shows that many of the nurses who took this postgraduate preparation did, in fact, go on to earn bachelor's degrees; some continued until they had earned master's degrees.

In later years this kind of arrangement for combining academic work with employment as professional nurse came to be known and used in many centers as the Learn-Earn Plan.

At the time of its origin, in 1932, the success of the idea had three equally important effects. At one stroke it removed the nurse from the rolls of the unemployed, restored her to self-esteem as a worker, and encouraged her to continue with professional preparation. Few adjustments to the emergency conditions of the depression can have worked so deftly to accomplish significant social goals.

For the instruction of the group of nurse students brought together in this way Miss Densford developed a procedure which had the further beneficial effect of bringing experts to her faculty. Any associated hospital which was willing to pay $200 a month for a qualified teacher might have her. The director and faculty of the school, drawing on their wide knowledge of womanpower, made the selections.

Everyone profited by these arrangements. Hospitals were better staffed than they had been before, in part by graduate nurses of a high type for whom they paid almost nothing. The profession gained in that the level of training in the clinical fields was conspicuously stepped up. Individuals benefited not merely by being restored to responsible positions in society but by improving their professional and educational status in a way that might not otherwise have been possible to them. The depression whose ways with the many had been so harsh showed to these few, at least, a curious flexibility in dealing with human problems. But this was true only because educational leaders like Miss Densford had known how to transform disaster into opportunity.

One appointment made on the basis of Miss Densford's plan proved to be of particular importance to the development of programs in nursing education at Minnesota's school. It brought to the Midwest a young woman whose background of preparation was as unusual as were her own resources of creative imagination. Myrtle Hodgkins (she later became Mrs. John Coe) has exercised a pervasive influence on trends in nursing and has added much to the effectiveness of instruction not merely in the institution of which she is a faculty member but to the current practice of the profession.

At the Classical High School in Providence, Rhode Island, the principal had said to the incoming class of which Miss Hodgkins was a member: "Any one of you who hasn't every intention of going to college had better leave *right now.*" She did go on to Pembroke College in Brown University, not because she was intimidated by the rigorous outlook of this Roman father, but because a cluster of interests had already filled her responsive intelligence with demands for more knowledge. These interests drew her now toward missionary service, now toward mathematics, and again toward medicine. The problem of which direction to take had not been resolved when, just as she was about to earn her A.B. at Brown in 1924, she went to hear a lecture given by Major Julia Stimson of the army school of nursing. Recruitment was ever at the back of the major's mind and she made personal appointments with several prospective students. In the course of her interview Miss Hodgkins said unguardedly that she had been "thinking of medicine" but that perhaps she would have to "come down to nursing." In a ringing voice the military authority of which became famous throughout the world to nurses, Major Stimson echoed the words: "Come *down* to nursing!" She would have the young woman understand that nursing was one of the noblest, as well as one of the most useful professions in the world. It was a lesson Miss Hodgkins learned promptly — and for life. The final result of the interview was that she enrolled in the army school. It served the purposes of an ambitious young woman well, for, even in that day the school's curriculum included public health and psychiatric nursing.

After earning her diploma in 1927, she joined the corps and became teaching supervisor in medical nursing under the farseeing directorship of Mary Tobin. It was during this experience that she developed the outlook on nursing instruction which enabled her to make many valuable contributions. Texts in the field identify her as "the first clinical instructor." This historical distinction Mrs. Coe wears today with the casual air of a woman who is more interested in the future than in the past.

Mrs. Coe's belief in the importance of clinical instruction was once set forth effectively in a paper read before the annual session of the National League of Nursing Education held in San Antonio, Texas, in 1932. It is the point of view of those who have worked, during the past quarter of a century, to broaden instruction in the clinical area, that formal classroom preparation is not enough to equip the nurse for her duties. There she learns "isolated facts." The " power of transfer" should not be counted upon exclusively to carry this knowledge over into "practical application." As Mrs. Coe said:

We are apt . . . to say that the ward is the laboratory where the student nurse applies the theory that she has learned in the classroom. But into what scientific laboratory would a school send its students with no other direction and assistance than the knowledge gained in lecture hall and reference library? And yet how much more important it is for student nurses to have competent and constant instruction in their clinical experience where their laboratory material is human life? It seems to me that our attention must swing once more from the classroom to the ward. We have taken it for granted that the student will absorb every detail of knowledge poured into her ears by six or a dozen instructors — knowledge entirely new to her at the time when she is making an adjustment to a completely different environment and new way of living . . . The ward has been a laboratory without an instructor; the student has been left to experiment by trial and error . . .

Having diagnosed the lack, Mrs. Coe assumed the task of filling it. For five years she functioned in the army school as ward instructor. Then, in 1932, because of the heavy pressure of economic circumstance, the enterprise which had been inaugurated by Dean Annie Goodrich and conducted later by Major Stimson with distinguished success was forced to end its history. Katharine Densford, determined as always to elevate the quality of instruction in the School of Nursing at Minnesota, was at that moment on the lookout for a new faculty member to institute the new procedures of clinical instruction for the benefit of her students. So she brought this original explorer of the field to Minnesota.

Mrs. Coe (still Miss Hodgkins at the time) was established at the Minneapolis General Hospital where, under the arrangement already described, she was paid by the city but was officially an instructor and supervisor of the University of Minnesota School of Nursing.

The way of the innovator was not easy. The new procedures had many aspects that baffled head nurses and administrators whose own training had been of the traditional kind. Indeed, all the circumstances of instruction were different from ones that had existed before even in her own broad experience. Under the Minnesota plan Mrs. Coe was working both with beginning students in nursing and with graduate nurse students. Her first step in this new kind of clinical instruction was to arrange a series of orientation discussions which introduced newly assigned students to the special needs of patients on the ward. Then she proceeded to work with each student individually at the bedside. Finally, she met with small groups in ward classes. The material for these discussions was drawn directly from the day's work. It included reviews of such problems in anatomy, physiology, and pathology as were involved in the nursing of specific patients. It included also consideration of symptoms, laboratory findings, diet, and the art of nursing itself as these applied to particular patients. The whole proceeding was designed to correlate the nurse's previously acquired knowledge of theory with the actual instance of illness. It was designed also, in its over-all effort, to give nurses what John Dewey once called the essence of education — "the vital energy seeking opportunity for effective exercise." And as Dr. Dewey also said, the method helped to communicate to workers a nourishing and sustaining awareness of the "privilege of learning."

The ward classes were conducted, at first, in the only space that could at the moment be made available — a small bathroom in the quarters assigned to sick nurses. Around the bathtub the students grouped themselves as best they could, and over the washbowl Mrs. Coe hung her charts.

For a time these mystifying rites were watched by many of the hospital personnel with lifted eyebrows. But by a gradual evolutionary process a striking change came about. Utilizing her aptitude for mathematics, Mrs. Coe had been able to demonstrate even before inauguration of the program that the new processes of instruction could save both time and actual expense while they provide better care for patients. It was not long before a head nurse, in tacit acknowledgment of improvement in the performance of the day's tasks, said that she wanted the nurses on her floor only after they had completed the orientation series of discussions because they came to their patients with so much better understanding. Another head nurse reported her surprise at finding that she had praised the results of the program to a fellow worker in spite of the frequent inconveniences it caused to the nursing service. Patients themselves became aware of significant improvements in nursing care. And, finally, hospital administrators recognized the arrival of a new day by providing space for ward classes which was more adequate if less picturesque than the tiny bathroom had been.

A dramatic example of how important it is in patient care to have a company of nurses who are prepared to cope with the unforeseen came with the sudden epidemic of heat prostration which occured in Minnesota at the time when Mrs. Coe was developing the program of clinical instruction. During the first day of the crisis almost one hundred patients were admitted to the medical wards of the hospital, many unconscious from the effects of an unusual kind of collapse, many with temperatures so high that a thermometer could not register them. Each was spread out between bath blankets, his body doused with alcohol while electric fans, placed at head and feet, played over the surface. The community responded with spontaneous good will by sacrificing the comfort of many a household to send fans by the hundreds to the hospital. But it was nursing skill in carrying out the campaign of the doctors that met the emergency. Once more a system of instruction that stressed the ability to adapt knowledge to a new situation quickly had justified itself.

It may be said that the effectiveness of Mrs. Coe's effort in expanding opportunities for instruction sprang from her own conviction that the service of science is not merely a call to duty but a call to adventure as well.

Two of the teachers who helped to make the school's faculty conspicuous — both for their individual achievements and for the places they have come to occupy in the world of nurses — were products of its own classrooms. Cecilia Hauge and Mildred Montag have traveled far from Minnesota to their present assignments; each has reflected high credit on the quality of her preparation in each phase of the journey.

Cecilia Hauge was graduated in the class of 1929 and immediately joined the faculty. She served with it until the outbreak of World War II when she was chosen to go as chief nurse with the reactivated University Base Hospital, Unit 26. She became, later, chief of nursing in the European theater and hers was the first unit to move from North Africa during the invasion. She was succeeded as chief nurse of the base hospital by Myrtle Kitchell, another important alumna of the School of Nursing at Minnesota.

After the war Cecilia Hauge exchanged her army uniform for that of a civilian nurse once more and returned to the faculty of the school. But only for a short time was she allowed to stay. Her usefulness in public work was so evident that government service again summoned her and again she went, this time as Colonel Hauge, eventually to head the division of nursing services in the national office of the Veterans Administration in Washington.

This tall, vigorous daughter of the Vikings had been reared in the home of a doctor father, Melvin Hauge of Clarkfield, Minnesota. If ever a man committed himself wholeheartedly to democracy's doctrine of service it was this robust and genial Norwegian immigrant who was not only the community doctor but its mayor, director of its civic chorus, and animator of so many of its projects that his neighbors might have been excused for believing that he crowed the sun up in the morning. From this background Cecilia Hauge seized the qualities that have made her, too, an inexhaustible leader.

Another valuable faculty member of the 1930's was Mildred Montag. She also brought to the task of teacher in a school of nursing the unusual kind of preparation that Miss Densford asked of colleagues. Before entering the School of Nursing, Miss Montag had been graduated from Hamline University with a major in history.

For two years after her graduation from the school Miss Montag served on its faculty. Subsequent experiences have led her to Teachers College, Columbia, where her work as teacher, writer, and consultant with other educators has given her an important influence on current trends in nursing. She has been, in particular, a major figure in the work of developing the two-year programs in nursing education now offered by many junior colleges.

Many more such teachers of unusually broad background joined the faculty in response to Katharine Densford's urgent call. Frances Lucier's personal history presents another interesting variation on the theme of how the modern nurse comes by her preparation. The early years of her college career were spent at the University of California, where she planned to become a teacher of Latin and French. But nursing proved to have the same kind of insistent attraction that it had for many young women of her type. She was graduated from the Minnesota school and had experience in two hospitals before marriage took her to Chicago. Thereafter the curious rhyming of circumstance led her many times across Katharine Densford's path. The first meeting occurred when Mrs. Lucier applied for an assignment in the Cook County Hospital and its assistant dean, Miss Densford, received so widely experienced a young nurse with gratitude. Later, a change of her husband's business base brought Mrs. Lucier back to Minnesota where Miss Densford was now director of the School of Nursing. This time the reunion proved to be a permanent one. On various part-time and full-time assignments Mrs. Lucier has been conspicuously associated with the development of nursing education at Minnesota for more than two decades. During World War II she was acting superintendent of nurses and has been, since 1945, instructor in the school and assistant to the director.

During the depression, the reputation of the school as a progressive institution enabled it to attract many women who became valued members of teaching's womanpower. Ruth D. Johnson came to Minnesota shortly after the closing of the army school where she had been Mrs. Coe's colleague; she remained in Minnesota until she was appointed assistant dean of the School of Nursing at Duquesne University. Later she became dean.

Julia Miller was another conspicuous figure of the period. She earned two degrees at Minnesota: B.S. in education and M.A. in educational psychology. When she left in 1943 she carried the indirect influence of the school far: first as creator of a nursing education program at the University of Georgia, then as an executive of the National League of Nursing Education (later the National League for Nursing), later as dean of the University of Arkansas School of Nursing, and finally as nurse consultant on an important mission to India.

A final note on bounty from the depression's golden hand must be added. During the poverty-stricken 1930's university communities enjoyed one important compensation. If the idleness of many people created nothing else, it at least created time — hours innumerable, which could be used by people who knew how to use them.

Research men never before had had time enough to accomplish what was on their minds. Many a project in which an investigator was interested had been filed under abandoned hopes for want of staff with which to carry it through.

Fortunately there were men in the government of the United States who were alert to the possibility of matching men and jobs. Officials of the Civil Works Administration (later, the Works Progress Administration) assigned, from the rolls of the unemployed, workers to serve as assistants, clerks, survey-makers on any university projects which could be activated promptly. Professor Maurice Visscher of the University of Minnesota has said that many investigations of cancer, just beginning at that time, could not have been completed without the support of the WPA staff. It was, in the words of Vice-President Malcolm Willey, a kind of "golden age for research."

The School of Nursing claimed a share of these workers. Miss Densford put them immediately to work on investigations of the kind for which she as one of the most articulate of leaders in the National League of Nursing Education long had been begging: time studies, evaluations of technique, comparisons of curriculums. Only a few years before writers for the professional publications had spoken of such efforts as though they must wait for the leisure of a distant day when millennial conditions had come to exist. Instead opportunity had come from the depression. If the door had opened on Utopia only the slightest way, still there was a chink through which to admit the light of the future.

9

A Director Looks at Deans

🐾 ANOTHER major concern of the early 1930's, reform of the curriculum, required almost as much resourcefulness and ingenuity as did the problem of building up a strong faculty. In choosing teachers the director could work almost alone; but in revising courses of study she became involved in endless consultations with many others, all of whom had lively, and not necessarily congenial, ideas. Though it was appropriate and desirable, for the cooperative purposes of a university system, that there should be full discussion of changes, this wrestling with ideas seemed sometimes to achieve only deadlock. Meanwhile, problems showed their familiar mercurial tendency to elude decision.

Again the conditions of the depression complicated every effort. In a time of stress it seemed necessary to some advisers to discourage radical proposals for reform when here they ran against tradition or there darted up the blind alley of the budget. There were other collisions with the firm minds of university administrators. This last difficulty was the most baffling of all because Miss Densford had to deal with the disparate attitudes of two men who presided, as co-deans, over the affairs of the medical school.

Each of these matters can be most conveniently considered by itself.

Despite the fact that nursing had had, from the time of the World's Columbian Exposition of 1893, vigorous and highly articulate leadership, basic tradition with regard to training had changed slowly. Pioneers like Mrs. Robb had not regarded themselves as guides of a revolution in method. They had assumed that the fatherhood of the hospital represented an authority that must endure forever. Even the appearance of the university school had been hailed as progress chiefly because it put a mantle of academic respectability around the profession. As the old leaders saw their job it was simply to improve the tactics of preparation, not to change them fundamentally.

But, as nursing had moved into full professional status, a movement was begun, with the energetic support of the National League of Nursing Education, the purpose of which was to bring about radical improvement. What the new leaders wanted was a training program, rooted in science, and administered by teachers who had been scientifically prepared for their work.

The first step was to make a thorough survey of conditions in the field of nursing, past and present. A committee on the grading of schools of nursing was created by the profession itself, made up of representatives from the three important nursing associations, the National League of Nursing Education, the American Nurses' Association, and the National Organization for Public Health Nursing. Other members of the committee were drawn from the American Medical Association, the American College of Surgeons, the American Hospital Association, and the American Public Health Association. To the group were added also educators from the general field and representatives of the public. The work was financed in part by outside sources, in part by nurses who raised among themselves $115,000 during a five-year period. Dr. William Darragh served as chairman of the committee, and Dr. May Ayres Burgess, a trained analyst and statistician, conducted the survey.

Actually the investigations stretched over more than seven years, from 1926 into 1934 when the final report appeared under the title, "Nursing Schools Today and Tomorrow." Nothing could have been more detached, clear-eyed, and realistic than Dr. Burgess's summing up of the exhaustive study; nothing could have been more startling in certain of its revelations; and nothing could have had more profound effect on the development of schools during the following ten years.

Dr. Burgess pointed out, first, that there had been, in the early years of the century, an enormous improvement in hospital care. Under the influence of dedicated women like Mrs. Robb, hospitals themselves had been virtually remade. Patients no longer feared them as in the past they had done. Sickness transferred its base from the home to the hospital.

Then a curious cycle of events changed the outlook. The survey states the problem:

Because students of nursing were so superior to untrained attendants [who had previously made up the hospital staff] it was believed that "the way to have good nursing was to have a school." Student nursing improved the hospital service and, with the improvement, came greater demand on the part of physicians for more hospitals. With more hospitals came demand on the part of superintendents of nurses for more students. With more patients in the hospitals and more students to care for them there shortly resulted larger graduating classes of trained nurses with fewer [private] patients left for them to nurse.

This pyramiding of effort had produced a great surplus of nurses. As one report estimates "there was actually one [trained or untrained] nurse per 416 persons."

But the imbalance between supply and demand was only one bad feature of the situation caused by the too rapid increase in the number of schools. Superintendents, supervisors, head nurses all became swamped with work. Preoccupied by immediate problems, such people were unable to keep in step with scientific advances. Worse than that, their lack of capacity for leadership became depressingly evident. Hasty appointments to fill pressing needs resulted in the elevation to important jobs of mediocre women. The schools began to "lose the old traditions. Mediocre directors admitted mediocre students" and the alternation of pressures, first from the medical profession, then from the public, had the effect on hospital administrators of encouraging them to allow standards to be depressed more and more.

The situation at the beginning of the 1930's was, as Dr. Burgess saw it, "dark indeed." There were some 2,200 schools of nursing, the great majority of which were run by hospitals. Their purpose, quite unapologetically acknowledged by themselves, was to provide a supply of nurses to do the work at modest cost. Students were still required to satisfy no such standards of preparation as other professions required of their beginners. Sixty-five per cent were high school graduates; twenty-seven per cent were not; only seven per cent had had work in college; only one per cent had finished college.

The result was that nursing had deteriorated. There were too many entrants into what must now be called an overcrowded field. The depression had aggravated the situation by creating a "new poor" with no money in its pockets to pay for nursing care. But actually, a critical situation had existed long before 1929. Many a nurse had been unemployed for the greater part of her professional life. Yet in the midst of this surplus there were far too few able administrators. Women bearing great responsibility "struggled along with pitifully inadequate background." To this catalogue of lacks Dr. Burgess added more. There was a dearth of nursing literature — little about techniques, next to nothing about hospital administration. As for research, it was "virtually unknown."

It was, the survey pointed out, the job of the university schools to do something about a steadily worsening condition. They alone had facilities for filling the gaps; they alone could exercise the influence that would give standards another upward thrust. Upon them lay the responsibility for supplying leadership. But to do all this they would have to improve their own programs.

With this uncompromising judgment, Katharine Densford was in complete agreement. Though the outlook at Minnesota was better than in many another school, it was still not good enough. For one thing, too little time was being spent in the classroom. As Miss Densford pointed out: "It would seem that a curriculum having only 852 didactic hours in a total of 7778 hours is rather meager in class work. A curriculum devoting but eleven percent of the student's time to class does not seem to me to have the correct balance."

To this Dean Lyon offered his emphatic: "Hear! Hear!" Hercules, still spinning among the maidens, produced no fine-spun theories about their future but rather the most blunt and realistic of judgments about their present situation. It was his frequently reiterated warning that though "nursing had, here and there, received university recognition" the claim could hardly be made for it, on the basis of the content of existing courses, that it deserved high credit. "By no stretch of the educational yardstick," he said, "can one make the present nursing curriculum merit a college degree. Nurses are highly trained in manual skills; they are not broadly educated."

The ideal place for training nurses, he once told a convention, would be "a fairly large school organized under an existing medical school or college which possesses a good scientific faculty and equipment. Only there can the standards of admission, teaching, examination, and graduation, found in higher education, be assured. Only by such organization can it share existing facilities such as laboratories, libraries, collections of illustrative material and teaching forces needed for good teaching. Only thus can nursing education be integrated with other education."

With this kind of encouragement Miss Densford began to create an atmosphere in which "proper university work" could be done by candidates for the degree. In 1932 she and the faculty of the school asked the University Committee on Admissions for advice in the selection of students. An outgrowth of this request was an important study of the criteria for selection made by Ruth Merrill, under the direction of Dr. Harl R. Douglass. Her doctoral dissertation set forth its findings. In the course of this study batteries of pre-entrance tests were administered to successive entering classes. The result of turning such searchlights on the problem of high mortality was that failures in the first quarter decreased markedly. More careful selection helped the hospital as well as the school, for as Miss Densford's report observed it was no longer necessary "to house poor students during the first phase of training only to have them drop out when they had just begun to be useful in the care of patients."

Many new opportunities were opened up to the five-year students. In the field of psychology they took not merely the required introductory course but were urged to choose, from many electives, other subjects that touched closely on their work. Dr. Richard Elliott cooperated with Miss Densford to draw her students into such courses as Introduction to Laboratory Psychology and Psychology Applied to Everyday Life.

The department of sociology was equally hospitable. During the depression Dr. F. Stuart Chapin was vigorously active in the university man's chief task of adapting educational programs to existing conditions. He converted a chaos of idleness and fear into a communitywide laboratory for the study of social problems, requiring his students to contribute to the alleviation of misery through internship in the various social agencies of the Twin Cities. His success was so striking that his school of social work, now established as a separate unit within the arts college, became one of the best known and most influential in the country. Students in the School of Nursing were required to take such of its offerings as the course in Social Pathology.

Dean Lyon's desire to see the creation of a pattern of nursing instruction which would be closely integrated with the large pattern of a liberal education was gradually being realized. The essential idea of a university system — all for one and one for all — was not merely acknowledged as an ideal; it was put actively to work.

At the same time all courses for graduate nurses were revised by Miss Densford and the faculty to broaden the range of clinical experience in public health nursing fields. Divisions of the university whose work was closely related to that of nursing opened their doors. Child welfare admitted nursing students to its courses. So also did the department of public health.

This emphasis on the rights of the degree students and of those enrolled as graduate nurses was entirely deliberate. More and more of the applicants for admission to the School of Nursing asked for the five-year program. But the great increase in their number was not the chief reason for this special attention. Dean Lyon and Miss Densford agreed that the three-year plan should be dropped as soon as possible. It was difficult to train students on two levels simultaneously, particularly when diploma candidates and degree candidates had to share some of the same classes. Throughout the 1930's the influence of the profession was directed toward the full development of college programs in nursing education. This was the objective of the Association of Collegiate Schools of Nursing which held its first conference in 1933 and set up machinery for permanent organization in 1935. Its recommendations urged concentration on work of professional quality. And so it was that the proposals of the Minnesota school looked toward the gradual "withering away" (to borrow and sterilize a Marxist phrase) of the diploma program.

But while its students remained in the school their interests were given thoughtful attention. New opportunities were arranged for them. They were assigned, for limited periods, to service in public agencies — Visiting Nurse Association and Infant Welfare Society (later Visiting Nurse Service) in Minneapolis, the Family Nursing and Baby Welfare Association (later Family Nursing Service) in St. Paul. When the General College was opened, in 1932, to fill the needs of those who did not expect to follow a full academic course leading to the B.A. degree but were content with two years of post–high school study, students of the three-year program in nursing were encouraged to take its "overview" courses, dealing with general problems of modern living. Meanwhile Miss Densford used all of her gifts of encouragement and persuasion to lead diploma candidates of high ability into the degree program.

In the matter of financial support for schools of nursing Miss Densford and Dean Lyon shared the forefront in a campaign for progressive attitudes. Neither showed the slightest timidity in criticizing not only traditional practices of the hospital schools but those of their own institution. In her first declaration of war on the past, Miss Densford wrote:

The educational needs of the School of Nursing in the University of Minnesota have been completely submerged by the financial (that is, service) needs of the hospital and the educational needs of the medical student. This is true to a large degree in most schools of nursing. But probably no professional woman contributes more to community welfare than does the graduate nurse, giving, as she does, both bedside nursing care and positive health teaching. She merits a preparation which is as well-planned and as sound as is that of other professional workers. This involves, in the last analysis, the same kind of support. The university, from public funds, contributes largely to the education of the teacher, the doctor, the dentist, the pharmacist, the home economics worker and others whereas the student nurse not only receives little in terms of formal education but through her services she actually contributes to the financial support of the hospital.

She would not wish to suggest, Miss Densford went on, that the School of Nursing offered students "a garment with but a seamy side." Much in it was good. But much could be better. "For a wish to do better we may, perhaps, be pardoned in a university school."

Dean Lyon, to whom this statement was addressed, had no difficulty in pardoning her because he was in wholehearted agreement with her point of view. He, too, was concerned with the problem which he discussed again and again with nursing leaders, that of "getting the profit out of nursing education." This he believed to be the first prerequisite for making a new start.

A study, conducted at the Massachusetts General Hospital early in 1932, had shown that the institution made a very large profit on its nursing school. Dean Lyon's breakdown of the figures indicated that by her service each student contributed from $200 to $450 toward this profit. Working for reasons of convenience and fair play with the lower figure, Dean Lyon estimated that each year the 80,000 student nurses of the country rolled up a surplus of $16,000,000, enough to support some 12,000 hospital beds. Each of these beds, he insisted, should bear a placard reading: "Supported by the Student Nurses of America."

They maintained them as surely as though their membership constituted a philanthropic organization.

This, Dean Lyon did not hesitate to say, was a "racket," one in which the then prevalent menace to society, Al Capone, might well interest himself. The dean spoke "roughly" of these sensitive matters because he wanted the hospitals to understand that they had "no moral right to the money student nurses earn." He wanted them to see that "this money should be used for the education of the nurses." He wanted them to acknowledge that "in the long run they would be better off if they trained the nurses better with the money students earn."

Before a session of the National League of Nursing Education, held in San Antonio in April, 1932, he flung a challenge directly at his audience. "Perk up, some competent personality in this gathering," he said. "Gather your confidence like a militant missionary. Sell to your trustees and superintendent the advertising slogan of a hospital that does not exploit its students and has affiliated with it the best school of nursing in America."

He did not have to look far to find a competent personality to act as missionary. At the same session of the League, Katharine Densford had been preaching the same doctrine. "We are not unmindful of the financial difficulty involved in any such program [as the ideal one she had outlined] nor do we hope for an immediate Utopia. [However] there are more than 2000 schools of nursing in the United States and some 7000 hospitals. If 5000 hospitals find money (in normal times at least) to care for patients, may not the other 2000 in the not too distant future do likewise?"

Happily Miss Densford was able in the course of her administration to achieve a steadily improved prospect for students in the hospitals of the university. Hours of assignment there were reduced in number from 48 to 44, then to 40, and later still to 30. The essential purpose was always to protect the rights of the nurse as student. Against compromises affecting educational opportunity Miss Densford took her stand firmly.

But it was a task for the crusader especially in the early years of the 1930's. The depression created major obstacles to reform. And there was also the difficulty that a certain difference of opinion in matters of nursing education separated the minds of Lyon and Scammon, the two men who shared the administration of the medical school.

The history of their co-deanship is in itself of interest. As the end of his regime approached, Dean Lyon developed the idea of establishing a pattern of organization which would integrate all phases of the work in the medical sciences in one large, inclusive design. Deans of schools of medicine, dentistry, pharmacy, and nursing would report to an overall dean of medical sciences who, in turn, would report to the president of the university.

For the post of super-dean, Lyon nominated his former colleague who had lately gone to be dean of the division of biological sciences at the University of Chicago. Scammon was to be the dean of medical sciences while Lyon himself would continue to be dean of the medical school.

Early in his career Dr. Scammon had established himself as a genuinely original intelligence in the field of research. His studies of growth were searching and complete. Many years after Scammon's work was over, Dr. Ancel Keys said of his investigations that they stood solidly in the foreground of scientific thought after many years of further study, unaltered in any essential way by new discoveries. He was so brilliant a teacher that students spoke rhapsodically of his blackboard diagrams as though they were in themselves works of art like the sketches of Leonardo.

Scammon had a pair of dark eyes that seemed in the most casual glance to reflect a lifelong habit of penetrating deep into mysteries. A walrus mustache bobbed with fascinating rhythm over a mouth that seemed unable to utter a sentence that did not contain either positive wit or its negative feature, a teasing irony. His bulk was enormous but he seemed to fancy himself as a sort of outsize gadfly to complacency. "The status quo," he used to say with the scorn of one who slammed a door on a charnel house. "No imagination!" was his charge of deepest contempt.

Dean Lyon's plan was never carried through to full development. Professional loyalties in some divisions worked against a proposal which seemed to them to threaten independence. Scammon's responsibility resolved itself into a kind of not altogether easy partnership with Lyon in which neither relinquished the lion's share. Their divergence of opinion was nowhere more apparent than in the relationship of each to the School of Nursing. Though Lyon had offered himself as champion of the nurse's right to an unencumbered share in the privileges of a student in a university system, Scammon took a different view. "During the depression," he frequently told the director of the School of Nursing, "it is your job to supply the hospital with nurses."

Yet they continued to work together until 1935 when they ended their administrative activities simultaneously, Lyon to retire and Scammon to accept a Distinguished Professorship of Research.

So, in the matter of budgetary reform, depression and later World War II slowed the progressives down to marking time. Meanwhile they turned back to the problems that could be handled independently, those of redesigning curriculums.

To the end of his life in 1936, Lyon's interest in the subject never wavered. In 1933 he served on a committee appointed by the Association of American Medical Colleges to make recommendations about their future programs to schools of nursing. His colleagues were Father Alphonse Mary Schwitalla, dean of the St. Louis University School of Medicine and Dr. A. C. Bachmeyer, then superintendent of the Cincinnati General Hospital, later Associate Dean in the Division of Biological Sciences at the University of Chicago and superintendent of Billings Hospital.

Their published report endorsed the enterprise of the university schools of nursing and urged them

. . . to bend every effort toward the safeguarding of educational standards by conducting them on a collegiate level . . .

. . . to elaborate educational programs not alone for the curriculum . . . leading to the degree of Bachelor of Science [but also for] advanced curricula in the various fields of specialized nursing endeavor.

. . . to encourage sound educational experimentation with special reference to the solution of existing controversies concerning curricular administration.

. . . to accept the principle that courses be formulated with the same seriousness and on the same collegiate levels as are demanded of accredited colleges of arts and sciences, particularly with reference to the curricular content, the diversification of courses, the sequence of courses, the quantitative evaluation and full requirements of courses and a satisfactory equilibrium between theoretical and practical courses . . .

It must have given Dean Lyon satisfaction, as he reread this handbook for revolution, to realize that the School of Nursing in his own university had long since broken over the barricades and in all these ways carried the battle briskly to the enemy, complacency.

Indeed, he did not hesitate sometimes to set aside his hopes for the future and enjoy for a moment, before the next battle, the contempla-

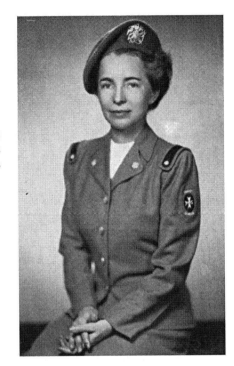

Lucile Petry Leone in uniform as
the head of World War II's
Cadet Nurse Corps

The University's base hospital in North Africa (1943)

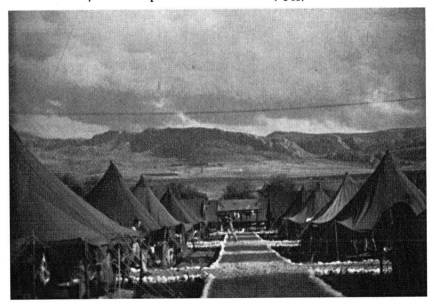

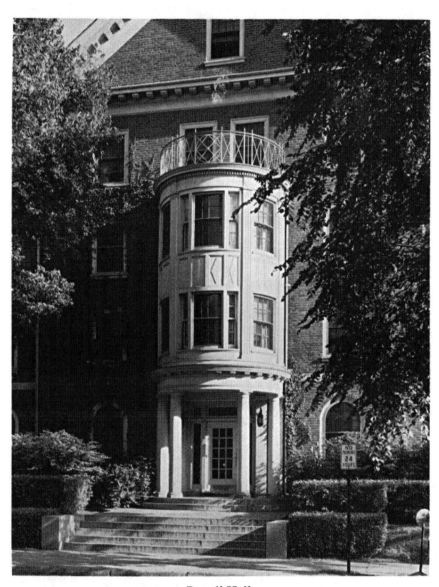

Powell Hall

tion of present achievement. For the *Alumnae Quarterly* he once wrote this tribute:

The students, alumnae and university may well be proud of our School of Nursing. Quite apart from the five-year curriculum which presents excellent features, it can be demonstrated, I think, that not in two percent of nursing schools of the country are the standards so high, the scientific instruction so thorough, the services so diversified and adequate as in our three-year course. All this the university is able to accomplish not only without expense to the state but with fairly considerable saving to the hospital in which the school operates.

At a session of the Minnesota Chapter of the American Association of University Professors, Anton J. Carlson once made a memorable declaration of independence for the teacher. "I don't look up to deans;" he said, "I don't look down on them; I just look at them."

During the first half of the 1930's, Miss Densford had had to show an unusual degree of that kind of independence. It was her job to look at two deans at the same time and yet not flinch. That she managed to look at them steadily and to come away from the encounter with benefits for the school — this may well be taken as the impressive measure of her success in the depression.

10

No Common History

Miss Densford's activities of the first half of the 1930's were not concerned exclusively with building up faculty and with reforming the curriculum of the school. No institution can be merely an organization created to fulfill a public purpose; it is also an association of human beings whose private interests must be regarded with a proper respect if the day's work is to proceed in an orderly and disciplined way. An institution which is part of a university system should be particularly attentive to all those matters which make incidental contributions to the task of spreading the advantages of a liberal education.

For far too long a time the liberal education of nurses at the University of Minnesota had continued to have conspicuously penurious aspects. The "healthy-looking crowd" of girls who had stirred the somewhat austere admiration of the board of regents, in 1919, had had a long line of descendants no less vital, no less educable. They had been asked to spend their days and nights in the same depressing, unsanitary setting of the scattered residences about which Miss Powell and Miss Vannier had vainly protested. The "temporary" housing arrangements seemed to have attained grim permanency.

Then, quite suddenly, in the depth of the depression an end to the situation came. The school was given its "hall for nurses" at long last.

"Tenacity of purpose" is the phrase that admirers of Katharine Densford have applied more often than any other to her character as administrator. Tenacity has seldom been so expertly balanced by tact. But it was always ready for service and not many hours passed in all of Miss

Densford's career when it was not applied to a purpose, with patience, with good temper, with a sense of sportsmanship — and with firmness.

To a woman who had always relished the pleasures of painting, music, and books (both as appreciator and as creator) it seemed entirely wrong that anyone should lack agreeable surroundings that made room for all these satisfactions. As soon as she arrived in Minnesota Miss Densford began to work actively for better housing. She presented the problem urgently to university officials, public men, alumnae of the school, friends of education — everyone who had an immediate or a general concern for the welfare of nurses.

However, just before Miss Densford's arrival in Minnesota, a discouraging succession of events had seemed to set back indefinitely hope for a new hall on the campus. In its 1929 session the state legislature had appropriated money for the improvement, but at the last moment friends of the School of Dentistry had succeeded in attaching a rider to the bill which gave priority to the project of building a new center for its interests.

A peculiar irony dwelt in this situation. To make room for the dentistry building the university must tear down several of the poor shelters which were all the nurses had. In the spring of 1931 they found themselves being evicted though no substitute residences were provided. Student nurses were expected to do still more doubling up though by now this must have seemed like an assignment for professional contortionists. The superintendent of nurses literally had no roof over her head. As the young women retired to their remaining "cottages" they must have listened with new loathing to the rats as they gnawed at shoes under the beds.

Into this crisis the Alumnae Association of the school now stepped almost en masse. Its members retained keen memories of the inconveniences of Grub Street and they were unselfishly determined that their successors in the school should have a better prospect. A committee of nine, headed by Minna Schultz Kief and including Anna Jones Mariette, was appointed to explore the possibility of getting action. Miss Densford, whose loyalty to the university was intense but who considered that in this matter it was the right of a democrat to speak up for himself, agreed that it would be proper for members of this committee to appear before the joint committee of the House and Senate of the legislature, acting on appropriations for the university. On a March day in 1931, they had their hearing.

Some of these gentlemen looked on with mild surprise as the alumnae vigorously put their case. "But we voted money for you two years ago," one of them observed blandly. "Did you, indeed?" retorted the spokesman, Minna Kief, and proceeded to give these absent-minded conscript fathers a brisk statement of the facts of life.

"What we ask," she said finally, "is a new appropriation which will be available immediately." *Now*, she suggested, would be just barely soon enough.

And her committee got it. It may have helped to make up the minds of legislators that representatives of the Minnesota Employment Commission were standing by to urge that there would be a good chance to put idle men to work.

Action this time was immediate. Before the year was over ground had been broken; dedicatory ceremonies for the opening of the hall were held in October, 1933.

All of the loyal friends of the school participated eagerly in making plans. Dr. Beard, long in retirement from the medical faculty but still the Nestor of nursing, kept a watchful eye on designs. When it was objected that certain suggestions would be out of sympathy with the prevailing architectural style of the "new campus," he blew the protest away with a pleasing display of his old-time authority. "The campus has every kind of architecture, known and previously unimagined," he said. "Let's have what we want."

What Miss Densford and the students got is one of the university's finest buildings, a triumph of conservative taste. Its Colonial façade is, in fact, completely in sympathy with the style of the nearby dormitory for men, Pioneer Hall. It presides over the neighborhood, with a quiet and welcoming air of dignity, at the end of a street bounding the medical center, near the entrance of the original Elliot Hospital. In front the windows look out on the whole area devoted to medical science activities; in the rear, the view is of a handsome stretch of the Mississippi. The E-shape of the building stands five stories high on the street side and reaches down, through seven levels, along the high terrace of the river toward its bank — a typical example of what has been called "Minnesota's subterranean skyscraper style of architecture."

In the beginning, before additions were made, there were rooms for three hundred students and space for their supervisors. A comfortable "great hall" and serviceable corridors must have tempted the bicycle riders of the old days to renew their skills. A tunnel joins the building to the hospital. Gone forever are the days of shivering on Washington Avenue while the trucks race by.

Everyone who should have been there was present for the dedicatory ceremonies in October, 1933. To the hall (not "home," a word, which to Dean Lyon's ear, seemed to hold an echo of the old "monastic, almost military" way of life which had held independent women in subjection far too long) came Miss Powell, Miss Vannier, of course, Dr. Beard and, with them, the president, the director of the school, and all the deans of medical sciences. Students listened with what they later reported to be filial pride as Dr. Beard gave the address of the occasion. There could have been no other possible sponsor in baptism of this new project, and Dr. Beard spoke the word of aspiration with unabated fervor.

"If it is true that 'Hope deferred maketh the heart sick,'" he said, "it should be true, in reverse, that the fulfillment of hope should give us a great and abounding joy . . . I am glad to think that the history of this School of Nursing is no common one. You must make the Nurses' Hall a part of it."

Miss Powell had her word later. Coming again to Minnesota in 1936 to give the Richard Olding Beard lecture, she presented a full, factual account of her stewardship, showing once more how sense and sensibility had presided together over her administration. Not a word of either self-adulation or self-pity (those occupational diseases of the unoccupied) was allowed to trickle through.

I feel great pride in what has been accomplished by my successors in the school. I am thankful for the close personal contact I had with faculty and students, for the fine team work we had with the medical staff and interns when we were all working for the good of the patient as well as for the education of students. One of the great compensations that has come to me since my retirement from active work has been the continued love and loyalty of all those students who graduated from the School between 1912 and 1924.

So she went back to Virginia to live another six years before she retired finally into history. She lived long enough to know that, in celebration of the school's thirtieth birthday, the nurses' residence had been renamed for her, Louise M. Powell Hall. This was the first time that the university had honored a living person in this particular way. And, surely, no one had ever earned distinction more soundly.

A curious effect of the depression on the School of Nursing is still to be noticed.

One of the underlying principles of Dean Lyon's campaign to "get the profit out of nursing" had been that hospitals should pay for their service instead of expecting to have it done by apprentices. During the 1930's they began to do so. The reason was one that had a tragic background. But improvements in principle, even if they enter a system covertly by the back door, must still be received with a certain gratitude. In a world where motives seldom are quite innocent of the impulse to seek personal advantage, those that work, even indirectly, to the advantage of everyone have their value.

During the 1930's, when wage levels fell lower every day, hospitals began to discover that they could afford to pay graduate nurses for the work that had been done previously by student nurses. And so, in a way, Dean Lyon's idea of the proper way for an administrator to set up his program was realized.

Now the need for the Central School began to disappear. The affiliated hospitals could supply themselves with staff from the lists of available graduate nurses and they needed students from the university no longer. Indeed, it became with each of the administrators a point of pride to help alleviate unemployment by giving their work to women who were already members of the nursing profession and who needed jobs.

The Northern Pacific Hospital was the first voluntarily to withdraw from the affiliation which had been set up in 1921. Its director suggested to the School of Nursing that the assignment of university students be discontinued after January 1, 1933. The board of regents approved "with the understanding that the hospital agrees to accept on a part-time basis a reasonable number of graduate students desiring to take academic work at the university."

The Miller Hospital took similar action a year and a half later. After June, 1934, with the exception of the period of World War II, no first-year students were assigned to it from the university. The Miller was staffed with graduate nurses and ward attendants. One link with the university remained. All of the students in the School of Nursing were assigned there for three months' experience in caring for private patients.

These breaks were effected in the finest kind of temper. Cooperation between the university and the Miller Hospital, and also with the General Hospital in Minneapolis, continued to be close. During the war the hospitals were to be more interdependent than ever before. But the system of the Central School had begun to undergo evolutionary change and was eventually to be completely eliminated.

In the academic year 1937–38, the director of the school took her first sabbatical leave, naming Lucile Petry to serve in her place. In company with her colleague, Cecilia Hauge, Miss Densford set out for the International Council of Nurses at London.

This was a great occasion marked by the appearance, as a chief speaker, of the founder, the same Mrs. Bedford Fenwick who had been Mrs. Robb's guest at the World's Fair of 1893. Complete with "huge feather boa," Mrs. Fenwick lent superb authority to the idea that women must work within the durable frame of world organization for preservation of the health of the human race. The ICN had been in existence since the turn of the century and its mission, followed with intense idealism and immense energy, had helped to put the profession some fifty years ahead of the rest of the world in global planning.

Katharine Densford's own interest in international relations among nurses had begun in 1929 when she attended the session of the ICN held that year in Montreal. Both her interest and her influence grew steadily. She served for a ten-year period as second vice-president of the ICN and her activities took her many times throughout the world in the service of the principle that all men everywhere must be enabled to share the benefits of science in health care.

America could have found no better representation than this tall poised woman who, in the years of her early maturity and ever thereafter, looked more like the classic representation of the Greek ideal of womanly intelligence, Pallas Athene, than even the most hopeful romantic had ever imagined a human being could look. To these immediately impressive attributes Miss Densford added a quiet humor, a habit of treating every fellow worker like a colleague worthy of exquisite courtesy, and a nurse's air of having the competence and energy to deal with any kind of emergency, great or small.

Over the years their sense of her quite unusual degree of self-mastery and mastery of circumstance has prompted women everywhere to draft Miss Densford for leadership. A catalogue of the public posts she has held suggests the wide range of her contributions. Lending her executive ability to local and national organizations of nurses as well as to one of world influence like the ICN, she has served as president of the Minneapolis Nurses' Association, the Minnesota Nurses' Association, the Minnesota League of Nursing Education, and the American Nurses' Association. She has been a trustee of the Harmon Association for the Advancement of Nursing, a member of the executive and steering committees of the National Health Assembly, a member of the Board of the National League of Nursing Education, a member of the National Commission on Hospital Care, a member of the special medical advisory group of the Veterans Administration, and a member of the Mayor's Health Advisory Committee of Minneapolis. Innumerable committees of the Red Cross, the Foreign Policy Association, and the National Association of Parliamentarians have had her active participation. Often she has served as faculty member of institutes arranged by such organizations as the American Hospital Association. She has also found time to contribute much to the literature of nursing. Articles have dealt with matters as highly specialized as the techniques of tuberculosis nursing; books with the broadest of concerns. Besides the work on counseling, done in collaboration with Miss Gordon and Professor Williamson (for which the authors received the first award in nursing literature made by McGraw-Hill), she is co-author with Millard Everett of *Ethics for the Modern Nurse*, a study which opens up long vistas of consideration for the professional woman in developing a personal philosophy.

The cumulative value of all this work has brought Miss Densford honorary degrees — that of D.Sc. from Baylor and that of LL.D. from her own university, Miami. Many organizations within her adopted state have offered her recognition of distinction. The Junior Chamber of Commerce in Minneapolis named her among the 100 Living Great of its community; Hamline University in St. Paul cited her as one of the twenty-eight outstanding women of contemporary Minnesota history; the Y.W.C.A. of Minneapolis chose her as one of the twenty-one woman leaders of the region. Her endless journey of discovery has taken her, sometimes on her own initiative, sometimes under the auspices of national and international organizations, around the world, across Russia, into Africa where Mrs. Albert Schweitzer became her friend, to Brazil, to Ireland, to Turkey, to Iceland, to China.

This has been, to borrow Dr. Beard's phrase, "no common history." It has made the director of the school, as an account of her career in her hometown newspaper once pointed out with pride and complete accuracy, "one of the most famous nurses in the world."

As she traveled across Russia in the summer of 1937, returned to America in the fall with Cecilia Hauge to enroll in classes at Teachers College, Columbia, and then set out again in the spring to study nursing in the world laboratory opened by a world tour, the director was constantly in communication with the base at home. Lucile Petry wrote six-page letters in longhand to give full accounts of the "situation in pediatrics," of the outlook for the budget, of the possibility of attracting funds from this, that, or the other outside source.

When Miss Densford returned to Minnesota in 1938 she may have reflected that the old order for the school was passing. Dr. Beard had died in 1936. Dean Lyon had retired in the same year and died a few months after. Dean Scammon had returned to the interests of research leaving to Dr. Diehl the work of leading the College of Medical Sciences into what proved to be a period of enormous productivity in service and in investigation.

The responsibilities of the director of the School of Nursing were both more exacting and more stimulating than ever before. The depression was wavering through various stages of recovery and recession into history. World events were prodding human society at the point of a bayonet and under the heavy blows of the truncheon, into another tremendous crisis. A new era was beginning and though the prospect for humanity was not good, it was one that offered opportunity for those who had accepted the job of alleviating pain.

11

Epoch of Responsibility

❧ THE world after 1938 became a battlefield not merely in the literal sense but for ideas as well. Two radically opposed philosophies began a contest for the possession of men's minds. Hitler, as he swaggered and bellowed his way into domination of the European scene, gave appalling utterance to one of these concepts. He claimed a right to impose on humankind a ruthless domination that took thought for no value other than that of establishing for the German people a dictatorial ownership of the earth. The methods by which this domination was to be achieved included lying, repudiation of compacts for international cooperation, torture, and bloodshed. A German historian has called the period that Hitler's influence brought to explosive fulfillment "the epoch of irresponsibility."

But not all people had been taught from infancy to lisp the rudimentary vocabulary of evil. In response to this kind of hysteria there developed, inevitably, in free minds exactly the opposite attitudes toward the problems of mankind. Nothing more reassuring with regard to the future of the race has happened in the twentieth century than the immediate retort to anti-humanitarianism that came from the democratic countries in the moment of Hitler's ascendancy. The answer was not limited to verbal eloquence though there was plenty of that when Churchill and Roosevelt entered the forum. The really significant thing was that active programs for the amelioration of human misery were instituted wherever the democratic ideal could spread its influence. The forms taken by this impulse to relieve distress are too familiar to require listing. In the policy of the United States government they ranged from the social legislation of the prewar years, through the lend-lease operations of the war period, to the Marshall Plan and subsequent measures for the aid of backward countries. What actually had happened was that civilization, to save face as well as to save its very existence, had undertaken to defeat Hitler's epoch of irresponsibility by inaugurating its own epoch of responsibility.

It is not a sentimental exaggeration to say that nurses, having a natural preoccupation with the forces of conservation, were peculiarly responsive to the challenge of this outlook. The maternal temper of the profession matured in response to new demands and developed new concepts of obligation which were summed up in phrases which were presently on the lips of leaders everywhere: "quality nursing" . . . "the total care of the patient." The history of Minnesota's School of Nursing, between 1938 and the crisis of Pearl Harbor, shows a consistent effort to follow this broad philosophy and to implement its purposes.

When Miss Densford returned to her desk in June, 1938, after her sabbatical leave, she brought an awareness of the world's emergency which had been alerted by her travels. She announced six objectives for the school. The first three had strictly to do with curriculum. Her suggestions were designed to avoid overlapping, to improve coordination, and to further integration.

The others were of more general character and had, from the standpoint of educational development, more significance. They were:

First, to give greater awareness of the need for understanding the normal as a basis for preventive and curative care.

Second, to emphasize the social aspects of all nursing.

Third, to develop a concept of nursing in which the student's practice becomes the functioning of social and scientific principles rather than the performance of techniques.

The implication of these suggestions is clear. The art of nursing had long since ceased to be merely that of making another pair of hands available to the doctor. Secure in the possession of a scientific background, the profession had developed principles and a philosophy of its own. But in the recent past this philosophy still had been concerned chiefly with the care of those who had fallen victims to disease. The job of the nurse was to move in and help repair damage already done. But now Miss Densford and leaders of her type urged that nursing must advance one step more — toward fulfillment as a social force. The task of nursing was not merely that of caring for illness; essentially it was that of protecting health.

At the same time Lucile Petry was reminding her students that the art of nursing "deals with human welfare." It must "emphasize the normal rather than the pathological." Its objective should always be "to procure for all workers" the greatest possible degree of "personal and professional satisfaction in vocational practice and daily living."

All leaders of the profession agreed. When Major Julia Stimson of the army school of nursing came to Minnesota in 1939 to deliver the Richard Olding Beard lecture, she told her audience of nurses that the hope for the future of their work lay in the fact that "scientists are proclaiming their belief that the discoveries of science may be applied more than they have ever been before to the welfare and happiness of the individual man." She asked nurses to think of themselves "as part of a vast army of those who are disseminating knowledge of health." With "their sisters around the world," she said, they "shared a united effort" to protect health as the inherent right of all men everywhere.

The mood of the epoch of responsibility was sympathetic to the desire of nurses to broaden their efforts as conservators of health. Lucile Petry returned from the convention of the National League of Nursing Education, held in April, 1939, at New Orleans, with the news that the real theme of the conference had dealt with the development, on a national scale, of a system of instruction all parts of which would be integrated in a large design. All the speakers on that occasion stressed the belief that nursing education deserved an important place in such a pattern. Dr. Earl James McGrath of the American Council on Education "seemed to take entirely for granted" that the training of nurses "must be included among the types of higher education." His fellow educators at the meeting were "convinced that the production of public health nurses is a proper function of higher education." Their discussions reflected the belief that "nursing and academic courses can be articulated in such a way as to compose a program meriting a degree and that clinical practice in nursing can be laboratory work in which high level intelligence operates in the application of principles to practice."

In short, the ambition of the nurse to function as part of a social force, serving human welfare in health as well as in illness, no longer seemed illusory to educators. Nor did it seem so to the government of the United States. Money, in addition to moral support, was being provided for the expansion of professional nursing service. In its leading editorial, saluting the prospect for the New Year of 1937, the *American Journal of Nursing* had called attention to the good news that an expansion of public health nursing had been "made possible under the provisions of the Social Security Act." This was an "event of far reaching significance" because "funds made available through the United States Public Health Service and the Children's Bureau of the Department of Labor" would result in "a tremendous increase in public health nursing services."

With the encouragement of all the agencies of a democracy, the nursing profession took a fresh look at all of its policies and functions, re-examined its programs and redesigned them in the light of what Miss Densford called "the social aspects of nursing."

One problem of human welfare to the re-examination of which the medical school and the school of nursing at Minnesota made important contributions was that of mental health. From time immemorial the subject had been wrapped up in mystery and shame. The tendency was to thrust it away into some dark attic corner of the mind, reserved for the insoluble, just as disturbed persons themselves were actually hidden away in obscure places. Only in the midyears of the century was the conscience of America awakened to the urgency of the problem. Then, at last, the subject was brought out into the light.

The opening, in April, 1937, at the University of Minnesota, of a new hospital unit for teaching, service, and research in neuropsychiatry was an event toward which the work of many years had led. As early as 1913 there had been discussions among the faculties of the university about the need for such a center of care and investigation. In 1923 the state legislature had gone through the motions of creating a "psychopathetic hospital" on paper but no funds for its support were actually provided. It was the persistence of Dr. J. C. McKinley that finally prevailed against "the law's delays." In 1935 he drew up plans and laid them firmly before the appropriations committee of the legislature. Already a distinguished man in his field (with Dr. Starke Hathaway he was later to work out the tests of the Minnesota Multiphasic Personality Inventory which became famous among investigators the world over), Dr. McKinley was able to persuade the members not merely of his own sanity but of his determination to satisfy a crucial need. He got his funds.

Station 60, as the new unit was called, could receive thirty-seven men and women. From among applicants for state care patients were selected with discrimination to make sure that students of medicine and nursing could observe various types of illness, those of organic as well as of functional origin.

Therapy was based on the hope of enabling the patient to readjust himself to the demands of society and to return quickly to his place in the community. He lived in a pleasant atmosphere of games, music, movies, parties, conversation, and all the activities of casual normal life. Looms, carpentry tools, and other equipment for the handicrafts were put at his disposal.

Each student in the School of Nursing now spent six weeks in the department. Her formal instruction in theories of mental illness went forward in close correlation with practice in nursing skills. As new treatments were developed by the university's research team, the student nurse watched their effect with firsthand intimacy. This constant association with investigators not only improved her art in the care of the sick but deepened her understanding of the role she would be expected to play in helping to reduce the number of cases of mental illness. As her teacher, Bertha Pritchett, frequently reminded her: "Many of the cases admitted each year to psychopathic hospitals could have been prevented by the education of parents, teachers, nurses and doctors in the application of the principles of mental hygiene . . . We cannot overstress the need of thorough courses in psychiatry in the general curriculum of medical schools and schools of nursing."

It was a thorough course which student nurses followed on Station 60. In addition to the care of their patients, they were required to have much field experience. They attended insanity hearings, watched the proceedings of the Juvenile Court, visited other psychopathic hospitals, and shared in staff conferences.

Just a year after the establishment of the psychopathic unit, another unusual opportunity for the study of emotional instability was opened up to students of medicine and nursing at Minnesota. Because its facilities for teaching in this field were considered to be good, the University of Minnesota was chosen by the Commonwealth Fund to receive a gift that encouraged further study. With additional assistance from the Home for Children and Aged Women (later Stevens Square), in Minneapolis, the board of regents was able to authorize the creation of a psychiatric clinic for children. Again, the result was to stimulate an interest in a kind of nursing that was designed to catch and cure mental difficulties at their beginning instead of allowing them to reach flood tide in an adult's sea of troubles.

By the end of the decade the School of Nursing had brought together for its students a rich and varied experience in pediatrics. The Institute of Child Welfare had made available the services of graduate students who conducted courses in phases of child psychology. The University Nursery School cooperated by assigning one of its graduate workers to part-time duty in the pediatric department of the hospital. Her job was to throw the light of expert knowledge with regard to the normal child's emotional behavior upon that of the sick child. Nurses also attended sessions in the Nursery School itself to observe its practices. Finally the out-patient department was explored by the school faculty to integrate experience there with clinical experience in the wards especially in matters dealing with children.

Now that training for the specialist had been accepted wholeheartedly by educators and government alike into the realm of higher education, Miss Densford was more than ever determined to attract into her faculty women with superior qualifications. She wanted teachers who possessed not only inherent ability but ones who had chosen to follow exacting academic disciplines before becoming nurses. A degree from a good college, plus a degree from a good school of nursing — this promising combination in a prospective faculty member was what she looked for persistently. Knowing the resources of womanpower in the field of nursing quite thoroughly, she did not have to look in vain. In 1939 she found this ideal meeting of personal abilities and professional preparation in Ruth Harrington.

This young woman had, in undergraduate days, allowed her imagination to explore widely through the possibilities for a useful life. Born in Brookline, Massachusetts, she had entered Radcliffe College and taken her degree there in 1929. Her major had been languages, but, along the academic way, she turned as often as possible to encounter Harvard's brilliant figures in the world of literature and criticism. She would, she thought, probably become a teacher of languages. But as she surveyed her past experiences she discovered, quite unexpectedly, that she wanted more than anything else in all the world of prospects to become a nurse.

There was a background for the development of this sense of vocation. Miss Harrington had been born — one of seven children — to a father who was himself one of eleven. Health, in this group, was not cherished as a value of family gospel; it was claimed as an inalienable right. It had shocked Ruth Harrington, when she went as counselor in a summer camp during vacation from college, to discover that this right was denied to many children of the Boston slums. When she began to think of a career there seemed to be no better one than that of undertaking to do something about helping to restore that right to the many.

After completing her basic nursing education she became instructor in a succession of hospital and college schools, never going far out of her native neighborhood. (There was still plenty of work to be done in Boston as she discovered in assignments at Simmons College and the Massachusetts General Hospital.) Wanting more advanced preparation she went to Teachers College, Columbia, where she took her master's degree in 1938. Minnesota had need of a substitute for Lucile Petry, during the spring quarter of the following year, and Miss Harrington accepted the assignment. Her success had been so great with her classes in the West that Miss Densford wanted her permanently. Miss Harrington returned as instructor in the fall of 1939.

Her first assignment was to put to use certain funds that Miss Densford had succeeded in getting for the School of Nursing from the federal government. For many years Congress had been supplementing its original appropriations to land-grant colleges with special allowances that were intended to encourage teacher-training. In early days the College of Agriculture had had many of these and later the College of Education had had its proper share.

The Smith-Hughes Act and, much later, the George-Deen Act provided money for the preparation of instructors who, in turn, were to teach vocational subjects in the public high school system. It was appropriate that nursing, too, should have a part of these funds, for the tasks of the school nurse had become more exacting and varied each year. By a complicated series of administrative maneuvers the George-Deen funds went from Washington to the Minnesota statehouse, to the State Board of Education, to the College of Education which shared the wealth at last with the School of Nursing.

Over the next twenty years Miss Densford, Miss Harrington, and the other members of the faculty were to have many grants, not merely from the federal government but from other outside sources, to be used for the development of new programs in nursing education and administration.

Their early initiation, difficult as it was, enabled them to assume leadership in finding new ways of dealing with the problems of human welfare.

These early experiences also gave Miss Harrington a background for the development of unusual features in the master's programs in nursing education which she now directs. She learned, as a colleague has said, not to allow teaching to become "roombound." To her each student in these advanced studies represents a new chance to give society a creative contributor to its work. She helps each to plan an individual program of investigations which will develop her capabilities to the utmost. And this she could not have done were she not what she fortunately is — a woman of genuine cultivation, discriminating intelligence, and broad knowledge of her field — one who possesses a stimulating awareness that a professional worker must be, first of all, a citizen of the world.

In the midst of the broad planning for the future of the school, Miss Densford and her faculty were made aware, as the decade of the 1930's closed, that responsibilities of an immediate, and very exacting, kind had been presented to them.

World War II did not overtake the university community, as the first had done, in a condition of incredulous shock. This time, teachers had known that eventually the United States must enter "the battle to save civilization."

In October, 1941, President Walter Coffey reminded his faculties, in the regular family letter which he sent to every unit, that the university itself was part of the national defense program which had long since begun in Washington. The Burke Wadsworth Selective Service Act, voted by Congress in September, 1940, as the first peacetime military conscription law in American history, had significantly reduced enrollment in all colleges where men students predominated. Many faculty members were on leave to do various kinds of work for the government. Long before Pearl Harbor the campus had been alerted to what its future must certainly be as a unit of a continent-broad defense encampment.

More than a year earlier the medical branches had been making concerted plans. On August 27, 1940, Dean Diehl was notified by the adjutant general that the Secretary of War had approved sponsorship of the Twenty-sixth General Hospital by the university. The man who had been a youthful interne with the Base Hospital, Unit 26, in World War

I was not responsible for its reactivation. An almost overwhelming response immediately settled upon him in the form of letters from volunteers for service. With the help of a committee made up of Dr. O. H. Wangensteen of surgery, Dr. McKinley of medicine, and Dr. Leo Rigler of roentgenology and radiology he selected a staff of officers. During February and March these appointments were made official by the adjutant general's office.

At the same time the staff of nurses was being selected by chief nurse Cecilia Hauge.

A Minnesota tradition of responding quickly to calls for service (it began at the outbreak of the Civil War when the state, then just two years old, had been the first to send emissaries to Washington with an offer to raise regiments of volunteers) found new expression when graduates of the School of Nursing, scattered everywhere, began to get into military uniform. Before Pearl Harbor many were writing to the *Alumnae Quarterly* to describe experiences at Fort Warren, Wyoming, at Camp Joseph T. Robinson, Little Rock, Arkansas, and at the Red Cross Training Camp, Bryn Mawr. And before the war was over an eighth of all the graduates from the school (since the year 1919) had seen active service of one kind or another. This was a startlingly high percentage considering how large a number must have been absorbed, long since, into the indispensable job of running households.

As the year 1941 moved on toward its dramatic climax, the School of Nursing mirrored in miniature dimensions all the strenuous activities of a nation ready to go to war. As had happened often before, Minnesota women were well out in front in all these emergency operations. Lucile Petry had taken leave from the university to go to Washington as special consultant to the United States Public Health Service under Surgeon General Thomas Parran. Her task was to help administer a fund appropriated by Congress to speed up the program of nursing education.

The hope was to put to work all inactive graduate nurses who could still walk the wards. The country had the greatest need of them.

At the same time Pearl McIver (class of 1919) became Senior Public Health Nurse Consultant and Alma Haupt of the same class became secretary to the Advisory Committee on Nursing Service of the Red Cross.

Under the spur of Public Law 146 which provided federal aid for nursing education, the university school stepped up all its programs. It was able to add to its faculty, establish refresher courses for the older graduates, create advanced curriculums, particularly in ward management, for recent graduates, and bring in new students by offering tuition, scholarships, and maintenance for young women who, without such aid, would have been unable to apply. No well qualified student, Dr. Parran said, should be "deterred from entering a school of nursing for financial reasons."

Then, in December, came the attack by the Japanese on Pearl Harbor. The shock for which the people of the United States imagined that they had long been braced came, nonetheless, with a shattering impact. Under this blow there collapsed also every theoretical notion held so stubbornly in the face of dictatorial vindictiveness, concerning an international code of honor between enemies. And out of the ruin rose up an image of total war as total irresponsibility, almost as total madness.

At Minnesota the president of the university was able to meet the emergency with a show of reserve which — could it have been more widely advertised — might well have frightened such hysterical men as Hitler and Mussolini. Walter Coffey had created for himself, as administrative official, a sort of special degree, Master of Crises. He had lived through many and he did not propose to be unsettled by this one. His regular letter to faculties, dated January 30, 1942, begins:

Since my last letter to you our country has become an active participant in the World War. Despite the fact that the United States was already launching an enormous defense program, the declaration of a state of war had a disquieting effect on the campus. I wrote to Governor Stassen pledging to him the willingness of the University, as an arm of the state, to do all it could to further the cause in which we are all involved. Ours is a common responsibility and we are sharing it willingly.

The aplomb of indestructible good will has seldom been expressed with more modest confidence. What Winston Churchill once called, with pride, "our British phlegm" had its counterpart in the temperament of many of his new allies.

The share of common responsibility taken up by the School of Nursing was to make a daily business of doing the impossible. Trained staff went into military service. Sixty graduate nurses resigned in a single day. The students took over their duties. Faculty members went into conspicuous places in public service. Volunteers for their posts appeared with unpredictable, almost unaccountable promptness, out of retirement.

Classes became larger and larger. In the academic year 1940–41 the total enrollment of the school was 750; in 1941–42, it was nearly 900. A special class of three-year students was admitted in January, 1942. A special group of college graduates was admitted, in June of each war year, to take an accelerated two-and-a-half year course. Faculty members of the School of Nursing multiplied their efforts and subdivided their days many times over. In addition to taking up the slack that resulted from the departure of so many colleagues into military service, they worked on innumerable committees in civil defense — local, state, and national. They helped to recruit the large company of students for which the United States Public Health Service was calling; even before the organization of the Cadet Corps they had succeeded in raising enrollment impressively. They allowed themselves almost no leisure at all but volunteered for still more tasks as instructors in home nursing; at odd hours of the day and night they met, for this purpose, with civilian groups of many kinds.

On the basis of highly persuasive evidence it may be suggested that few groups of American citizens took up quite so energetically the burdens of the epoch of responsibility.

12

Red for Courage; Gray for Understanding

◤ WHEN the federal government first undertook, as part of its defense program, to stimulate interest among young women in becoming nurses, its ideas of what would be needed in the way of financial support were comparatively modest. Like any beginner in enterprise — particularly in one that seemed to partake of a philanthropic character — Congress proceeded with a certain caution.

In 1941 a sum of $1,250,000 was appropriated to assist in nursing education. When this was found to be inadequate to maintain the projects launched in a first spurt of effort, a deficiency appropriation of $600,000 was added. In the year 1942–43, the figure was raised to $3,500,000.

By this time it had become evident to many that the job of producing nurses was no philanthropy but rather an absolutely essential war enterprise. It could not be supported by small appropriations. In the summer of 1943 Congress decided to go all out in a campaign to find and train the nurses, nurses, and yet more nurses for whom the services were calling.

It was a woman who discovered the formula for doing so. Representative Frances Payne Bolton of Ohio had been a civilian member of the board that governed the School of Nursing at Western Reserve University (later named for her) and she had a special understanding of the psychology of the profession. Put the young women into uniform and let them serve at the sides of their brothers in the army and navy, she urged.

So, the Bolton Bill was written, passed, and signed into law by President Roosevelt on June 15, 1943. What it created, with a bountiful appropriation of $45,000,000, was a new branch of service, the United

States Cadet Nurse Corps — the most colorful addition since the debut of the Marines. In the end the total cost of the program was $175,000,000.

The immediate response to the call for enrollment in the Cadet Corps proved Representative Bolton's wisdom. What young women had wanted, instinctually, was recognition of their group as one capable of moving forward, with the solidarity for which the nursing profession always had stood, equal in status with the men of the medical services, as they entered the theaters of war all the way from Africa to the South Pacific.

A glance at what had been happening to nursing recruits of Base Hospital, Unit 26, may serve to indicate how great an asset to military enterprise this passion for equality was. The chief demand of these nurses seems to have been that they be allowed to share all the discomforts, exactions, hardihood, and dangers of men.

Ever since she had resigned from the faculty of the School of Nursing to become chief nurse of the military hospital, Lieutenant Hauge (as she was in 1942) had been writing frequently to Miss Densford and her letters became a regular feature of the *Alumnae Quarterly*.

In January, 1943, she reported that the unit had landed overseas and the nurses were living "near a large city in small houses." They were going on long road marches in a "toughening up routine" but were "well fed on American rations." In February they had reached a land of palm trees (North Africa) and were living in a French villa. The nights were cold and the nurses had to wrap themselves in "everything available to keep warm" because there was no heating.

In March they were "living under field conditions." They equipped themselves "with men's shoes, coveralls, fatigue hats and leggings." They had become expert with tent ropes and stakes and had straw mattresses for their army cots. The girls "managed to keep in excellent humor." So much so in fact that they caught turtles, painted names on their backs, and bet on them in impromptu races. The boys thought it "more fun than a crap game."

In April they were on the road again traveling eastward under difficulties. They slept in their clothes night after night. One girl was injured in a jeep accident and died twelve hours later in Lieutenant Hauge's arms. The young women slept on the ground at night. But their morale was "never better." They have become veteran troopers. "Please don't misunderstand," the lieutenant urged. "I am not bragging. All I want you to know is that the 26th has not let the University of Minnesota School of Nursing down."

Insects were enemies as implacable as the Germans themselves. "The variety of beasties would astonish you . . . a nice centipede . . . a baby mouse in one bed . . . a luscious black spider . . . one nurse is on her head in her barracks bag right now looking for scorpions."

In May all that remained to be said was that "despite sand flies, sun and mud we have had a real adventure. The girls are all good sports and have shown ingenuity in improvising equipment for their tent wards. We find we can make anything we need out of tin cans and ration boxes."

Of such stuff soldiers are made no matter what the sex happens to be. As Representative Bolton had understood, student nurses wanted what graduate nurses had wanted before them: simply a reason to believe that they would be immediately and actively useful in war. A uniform would symbolize that reassurance.

Lucile Petry became director of the corps under the supervision of the Surgeon General. She had been on leave from the university since 1941. In 1943 she had resigned to become dean of the School of Nursing at Cornell. But without having actually served a day in that office she was given leave from the new post to serve in Washington. And as matters turned out she was never able to leave government work thereafter.

Never had the plan for the corps envisioned the establishment of a special school. Existing facilities were to be put to use, and of the 1,300 training institutions then in operation in the United States, more than half were enrolled in the program. This called for the acceleration of the usual 36-month course so that it could be completed in 30 months. Participants were given free maintenance, free tuition, and a monthly allowance beginning with $15 for the first nine months, and of $20 a month for the remainder of the period devoted to classroom instruction. For her last months of active practice the cadet entered either a government hospital or a civilian hospital during which time she received not less than $30.

In effect she felt that she was "in the army now" though in actual practice she was free, at the end of her training, to enter whichever of the services she elected. To do this she was morally bound. "In consideration of the training, payments and other benefits provided as member of the U.S. Cadet Nurse Corps" she agreed to "be available for military or other Federal governmental or civilian services for the duration of the present war."

All psychological considerations involving freedom of choice were discreetly and sensibly acknowledged. The pledge to serve throughout the war did not preclude the possibility of marriage. Many essential services, the first official announcement of the corps pointed out, including army nursing were open to married women. An increasing number of nursing schools were admitting married women. This acceptance of the realities of human experience showed how far nursing tradition had moved away from the monastic prejudices of the past. "Life must go on," as Lucile Petry knew — unlike Edna St. Vincent Millay who found herself likely, in times of crisis, to "forget just why."

This serviceable understanding of psychology supported Miss Petry in every phase of the corps' development. The best designers in the country were invited to offer suggestions for the uniform. In the long history of ritual and regalia men have given earnest thought to the importance of plumed helmets and scarlet jackets and it was no more than appropriate that women, joining their ranks with an equally brave display of hardihood, should have the best possible advice.

And the design proved to be good. Beginning with the idea that the cadet uniform must be symbolic of the qualities of the good nurse (red, for courage and inspiration; gray for serenity, mercy, and understanding) the creators achieved something extraordinarily attractive for those whose eyes, in contemplating young women, are not concerned primarily with symbolism. In winter the cadets wore gray wool suits, gray berets with matching shoulder bags, and reefer topcoats. In summer they wore gray and white chambray suits with gray felt bowler hats accented with red bands. Suits and coats bore scarlet epaulets and sleeve patches. The dignity of the corps and its insouciance both were well presented in this attire. The colors helped to diminish the drabness of war while the youth of the uniforms' wearers distinctly augmented hope for the success of their massed resistance. Conformity to a discipline, yet with a touch of jauntiness to it, confronted the stolid, dogged conformity of Nazi youth. The contrast could not but be reassuring.

An expert has described their insignia:

On berets and bowler hats was worn the historic emblem of the U.S. Public Health Service, the country's first humanitarian organization.

The design is that of the American spread eagle and shield superimposed on a fouled anchor and a winged caduceus. The fouled anchor symbolized American seamen in distress. The caduceus, sometimes called the Wand of Mercury, represents Aesculapius, the god of medicine and is the ancient symbol of physicians. The anchor and caduceus together represent the promise of medical care for those stricken while in the service of their country.

On epaulets and on patches worn on the left sleeve appeared another device, the eight-pointed Maltese cross. On the epaulets the number of crosses designated the grade of the wearer, one for a junior cadet, two for a senior cadet, three for a corps graduate. The eight-pointed Maltese cross was the emblem of the Knights Hospitalers of St. John in the First Crusade. Members of the original nursing-fighting order wore the cross embroidered on the left breast of their black robes of brotherhood. Each point of the cross represents one of the beatitudes of the Sermon on the Mount. The Maltese Cross has ever been the symbol of human compassion and life-giving skill.

Not until mid-July, 1943, were funds available for the enrollment of students in the corps. But since it was already in process of organization, July 1 has been fixed as the birthday of the service.

At Minnesota, as at all the other hundreds of bases, the moment gathered into itself many of the perplexities with which the profession had been plagued for years and then multiplied them by five. (This was the extent to which the student population of the school grew in the years of the corps' existence.) Where were the young women to be housed? Who was to teach them? How were they to be taught all that they must know in the abbreviated period of residence? What "instructional facilities" could be found to meet the challenge of numbers? How was the program to be accelerated without sacrifice of completeness?

To all of these questions Miss Densford found immediate, often highly ingenious, answers. The old problem of making do was a familiar one to her, and she met it, in its new guise, with the combination of professional knowledge, administrative skill, and housewifely adaptability which has always been required of the nurse.

During a hot July she went out looking for the promised land which, in fact, no one had promised her but which Washington simply asked her to materialize out of nothing. Housing for students was found with a readiness to improvise which shows what "the old lady who lived in a shoe" might have accomplished if only, like Miss Densford, she had been in possession of earned and honorary degrees from four or five universities. Members of the corps lived at home, with friends, in dormitories, in rooms rented for them.

Space for teaching huge classes presented an even greater difficulty. Miss Densford was almost ready to rent the dusty, but large, third floor of an unused building on Washington Avenue — scene of the school's first improvisations — when a bolder prospect for exploration opened up before her searching eyes. There in all its spacious splendor was the Cyrus Northrop Memorial Auditorium. She persuaded William F. Holman, professor and supervising engineer of the physical plant, to study the architect's drawing. On the third floor near the art gallery he found space that could be adapted to new purposes. The suggestion that it be turned into a nursing laboratory may well have startled Vice-President Malcolm Willey who had worked long and successfully to build up a distinguished center of the arts in Northrop. But the exigencies of the moment had commanding authority over other considerations and the order for conversion was given.

All through the war the nurses, in their hospital gowns and sensible shoes, carrying their stethoscopes and textbooks, streamed through Northrop, past the locked doors behind which the Minneapolis Symphony Orchestra was rehearsing under the phrenetic direction of Dimitri Mitropoulos. Up the broad stairs that led to the hall where once Thomas Mann had spoken, along the corridors where an exhibit of Matisse drawings might be hanging, the cadet nurses moved into the area where they learned to administer hypodermics and set up oxygen tents. Mitropoulos, Mann, and Matisse would have been the last to suggest that they were out of place.

The School of Nursing had responded well to the demands of the emergency. Indeed the success of the corps had been so distinguished as to deserve special commendation from the surgeon general.

In November, 1943, Dr. Parran sent word of his gratitude in a dramatic way. The scene was the Minnesota-Iowa football game. In President Coffey's box were Dean Diehl, Dr. J. F. Worley, medical director of the United States Public Health Services, the director of the school, and, in full uniform, Cadet Jeanne Larkin. Between the halves the president stepped to a microphone and spoke over a nationwide hookup. A telegram had just reached him reading:

Congratulations to the School of Nursing at the University of Minnesota for the magnificent effort it is making towards winning the war. You have enrolled in the United States Cadet Nurse Corps the largest number of students of any institution in the country. To make this possible you have greatly expanded teaching and housing facilities. The Cadet Nurses at Minnesota through their pledge to do military and civilian nursing are engaged in essential war service. My grateful appreciation to you, your faculty and students for your outstanding contribution.

The president publicly relayed this thanks to Miss Densford. It was a great day for Minnesota, one to which a certain measure of joy was added for President Coffey and Miss Densford, as well as the thousands in the stands, when Minnesota soundly trounced Iowa, 33 to 14.

It was one thing to enroll a huge army of students; to teach them was another. Miss Densford solved this problem by adding to the staff as faculty members twenty-nine graduate nurses who had volunteered for service.

Support for the work of the Cadet Corps was drawn from every available source. In October, 1940, Congress had passed the Lanham Act, empowering the president to identify and provide help for "particular areas" in which there existed "acute shortages of public works necessary to the health, safety and welfare of persons engaged in national defense activities." Miss Densford presented persuasive evidence that there was an acute shortage of space in which to house the army of nurses enrolled in the school. Officials of the Work Projects Administration promptly put funds at the disposal of the University of Minnesota for a broad extension of facilities. The thoroughness of these plans offers tacit testimony to the change in the status of the nurse. No longer did she have to beg for a reasonable amount of comfort. A new attitude found expression in the excellence of the quarters made available to her by provisions of the Lanham Act.

At the Miller Hospital, with which the university had new war ties, administrators acquired an apartment building and remodeled it into attractive rooms for 37 students. Then, on its own, the hospital built College Hall with accommodations for 60 more students.

The General Hospital added five floors to its building. Here 190 students were enabled to live in comfort and no one thought it an alarming abandonment to effete luxury when the rooms were furnished in good taste with modern chairs, sofas, and desks. One whole floor of the new residence was converted into classroom space, complete with nursing laboratory.

Best of all, a fine addition was made to Powell Hall. Besides living quarters for 170 students, its plan included an amphitheater for lectures and teaching, classrooms, a seminar room, and a laboratory. For the first time nursing classes were taught in rooms designed for the purpose. And, for the first time, nursing was given priority in assignment of space.

The annexes to the Miller were ready for occupancy in January, 1945; the addition to General was opened in February of that year; the enlargement of Powell Hall was finished in July. By that time D-day had passed, to be sure. But the gain to the university was permanent. Nowhere was there a whisper of complaint about wasted effort. The war had taught the lesson that today is gone and tomorrow is society's greatest asset.

In April, 1944, the scarlet epaulets of 684 cadets were flashing back and forth across the campus. The total enrollment of the school was at the thousand mark. The drama of this transformation called for public celebration.

On May 15, 1944, a demonstration of solidarity took place to which the word splendid may be unapologetically applied. It was the more impressive for the fact that all the conspicuous people involved in it spoke their minds with the simplicity and directness of civilians, not with the carefully rehearsed hysteria of the mass meetings in which the dictatorial powers were at the moment communicating their bleak intentions to the world.

The occasion was the first induction ceremony at which 96,000 cadets in various centers scattered about the country were received officially into service. By means of a national hook-up all were greeted at the same moment by the men and women who had been active in bringing them together.

At Minnesota the ceremony was held in the Cyrus Northrop Auditorium and participating with the university's own branch of the corps were those of many other units in the state. The total number was 1,500.

The young women in their gray and red uniforms marched four abreast across the mall with two lines of civilian nurses in blue work uniforms flanking them on either side. In the spit-and-polish perfection of their gear they were soldierly enough but, not being a military organization, they did not proceed with the precision that would be expected at West Point. To many observers the sight of them was moving precisely because these sober young women were young women still, not automatons who had been taught in their indoctrination as Nazi youth had been: "Don't think; obey." The cadets obviously were capable of thought as individuals. It was independence of judgment that had prompted them to put on these uniforms.

At the doors of the auditorium the mass formation broke and in single lines the cadets moved forward down the aisles toward the platform. As one of them remembered afterward: "We passed friends and relatives wondering if they could sense the sudden feeling of oneness that had come over us, the feeling that we were about to be recognized and sworn to positions we had chosen for ourselves, a newly unified body, awed and wondering . . ."

On the platform against the background of a huge Maltese cross sat the dignitaries of the occasion: the governor of Minnesota, representatives of army, air force, the U.S. Public Health Service, officials of the schools of nursing in Minneapolis and St. Paul, among them, Miss Densford. After an invocation given by Captain L. D. S. Foltz, chaplain at Fort Snelling, the director made the address of welcome. Tacitly Miss Densford recalled her own experiences of twenty-five years before.

"Always, in our nation's history," she said, "when there has come the 'hour of darkness and peril and need,' an aroused and listening people has heard, coming close after the young man's, 'I'll go,' also clear and determined, the young woman's 'I want to go as a nurse.' "

Presently the national broadcast from Washington began. It had been arranged by Captain Burgess Meredith and it testified well to a former actor's sense of occasion. Appropriate to the hour was nothing more or less than an expression of the folk wisdom of people who had become leaders chiefly because they were first of all workers, teachers, parents, contributors in the most direct and unpretentious ways to the well-being of the community.

Captain Meredith found exactly the right men and women to express patriotic fervor in terms of the next obvious duty toward humankind. He found them in Eleanor Roosevelt and Helen Hayes, embodiments for all the people of the United States of those profound values which abide in the simplest emotions. He found them in Representative Bolton, creator of the corps; the surgeon general, Dr. Parran, its organizer; and Lucile Petry, its administrator. He found another such representative citizen in Bing Crosby who, as a kind of universal elder brother to

American youth, had every right to be there and to dedicate a song to the corps.

Immediately after the broadcast, the cadets stood at attention to recite their pledge together. It was administered to Minnesota members by Pearl McIver, principal nurse consultant to the public Health Service. Governor Thye congratulated the corps; Lieutenant M. W. Eckel, chaplain at Wold-Chamberlain Naval Air Station, spoke the benediction; and the cadets marched out of the auditorium.

Just as university students have followed the tradition of wearing cap and gown throughout their Cap and Gown day, as they celebrate in small groups, so the cadets went about all afternoon in their uniforms. "Let's see you salute," a challenging young man of the services would demand from time to time. Then one of the more conscientious cadets would pause "to explain the civilian nature of the Corps and its non-affiliation with either the Army or the Navy." And the informal parade moved on. Shutters of cameras clicked whenever a corps member appeared; children's hands reached out to touch the bright sleeve patches; the temper of the day was good.

For many of the cadets it ended at sundown when they had to return to "five o'clock duty." They skipped hospitality at the free movie to which their uniforms entitled them and went back to work.

A similar ceremony took place on May 12, 1945, this time in the music building auditorium on the campus. In all 1,215 cadets were trained at the university. This was more than a twelfth of the total number produced in the whole country.

One way of estimating the value of an institution is to examine the use made of its facilities and of its personnel in a time of national emergency. During the war while the university school was training this army of cadets, the government at Washington kept drawing its teachers away to serve on special assignments. So also did the national organizations of nursing and the health agencies.

Ruth Harrington went on leave to serve as secretary for the National League of Nursing Education, on its special committee, Educational Problems in Wartime. She was elected to membership on the board of the League and served on many of its other committees concerned with post-war planning.

Thelma Dodds, assistant professor of nursing and director of nursing at Miller Hospital, went on leave to the Public Health Service as nurse consultant under Lucile Petry.

Other faculty members who entered the federal services to work in Washington, at Oak Ridge, and in various rehabilitation centers were Louise Waagen, Jean Taylor, Lucile Halvorsen, Caroline Rosenwald (Blanchard), Dorothy Sutherland, Pearl Shalit, and Rosalie Peterson.

Many of the school's women rose to high rank serving as chief nurses in hospitals, established all the way from the Philippines to Germany. Cecilia Hauge became its one colonel. Majors were Ellen Rasmussen, Hortense McKay, Georgia Nobles, Irma Block, and Irene Kemp. The group of captains was made up of Myrtle Kitchell, Beatrice Lofgren, Marjorie Sorenson, Cecelia Lediger, Harriet Grimes, Maida Hewitt, Gladys Saterbak, Anne Hauger Towey, Helen Walch, and Ellen Church.

This listing takes no account of the very large number of graduates who were made first lieutenants in the army and in the army air corps and lieutenants (j.g.) in the navy. Nor does it take account of the vast company of the anonymous great who, without expectation of receiving recognition of any dramatic kind, assumed the augmented work of those who took leave from their civilian tasks to enter the services.

Nurses of Minnesota wore their uniforms of whatever color with pride. They wore them also with distinction.

13

Toward Unity

🔊 AND now reconversion was the word. When the sternly concentrated effort of World War II was over and leaders in business, the professions, and the schools had their institutions returned to their private care, each organization had to be redesigned in fundamental ways. Industrialist, government official, doctor, lawyer, educator — all talked of "postwar planning." One underlying concept was common to the speculations of the late 1940's. It was evident to every thinking man that human society is an entity. Its parts are inseparable and interdependent. Planning must proceed with a proper recognition of this unity. Though infinity — the point at which parallel lines meet — might be the only haven in which mankind could hope to see its diverse interests finally reconciled, this must be the direction of progress. There could be no other.

The war had changed the outlook for every kind of project. It had shown that problems of previously unimagined proportion could be solved by cooperative effort. It had forced men and women to consider these problems in terms of their national and international implications. Whether that thinking was rooted in democratic principle or in the doctrines of communism, it was equally true that the world itself was the only unit which it was profitable to consider in making plans for the future. World trade . . . world government . . . world health were the phrases on everyone's tongue.

The somber realization that the development of atomic power would only aggravate the antagonism between the two philosophies — those of democracy and communism — left no one with the belief that the millen-

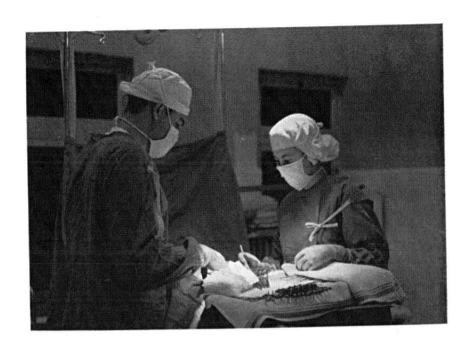

Nurses at work

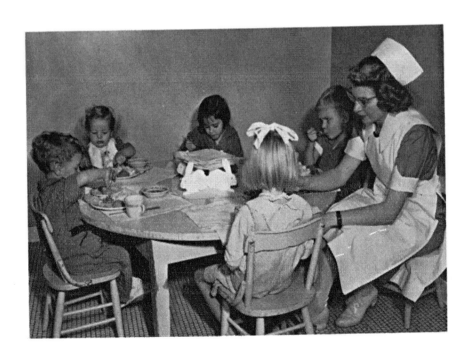

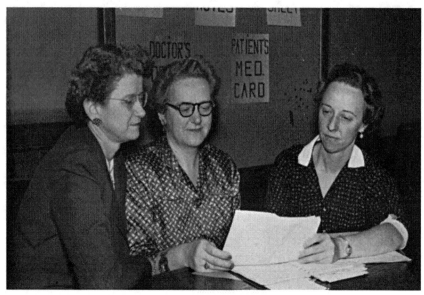

Margaret Grainger, Helen Goodale Florentine, Isabel Harris

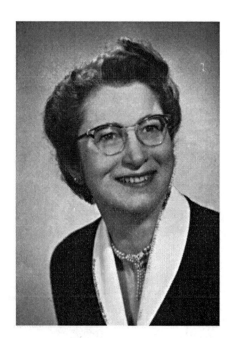

Myrtle Hodgkins Coe, first
clinical instructor

nium would shortly arrive. World trade and world government were fighting rather than soothing words. In these relationships there were no soft answers to turn away wrath. But when people spoke of matters having to do with the prevention and cure of disease the tone was different. The development of a World Health Organization proved their sincerity.

Dr. Wesley Spink of Minnesota, head of one of the large brucellosis centers of the world, found that, when scientists of different ideologies meet to consider the possibilities of making a common attack upon disease, they discovered more things upon which they could agree than simply the treatment of one physical affliction. Dean Athelstan Spilhaus of Minnesota's Institute of Technology, a tireless traveler in the interests of UNESCO, discovered that even Soviet scientists tended to drop their attitudes of guarded suspicion the moment they were able to talk to their fellow men, not as representatives of political groups, but as doctors or professors.

It was in the atmosphere of the laboratory that leaders in American education came together to discuss plans for the future. In her 1945-46 report to the president, Miss Densford observed that "Nursing education must offer scientific preparation that the nurse may the better understand and perform her functions. It must parallel scientific education with liberal education that the nurse may be socially, as well as scientifically, literate. It must avoid the waste of human resources and provide education in the real sense."

An important way in which a university school of nursing could serve the principle of unity in scientific preparation was to concentrate its attention on the requirements of higher eduction. The Minnesota school had continued until now to train nurses in the diploma program. This had been necessary during the war when the great objective was to achieve numbers. But, in normal circumstances, a sufficient supply of graduate nurses could be produced elsewhere. Nurses with advanced preparation must come from institutions that functioned on the collegiate level. It was to avoid wasteful duplication of effort that Miss Densford, her faculty, and the school's advisers wished to admit students to the degree program only.

In the course of its historical development the School of Nursing had followed the gradual progress of the University of Minnesota itself. In the pioneer period the board of regents had been obliged to accept whatever students presented themselves no matter how meager their preparation might be. At the start the so-called university had enrolled many pupils whose needs were rudimentary ones — instruction in "reading, writing, and 'rithmetic." But the first president, William Watts Folwell, had fixed his eyes — and with no ecstatic, visionary glow — on his ideal of the "genuine university." He had insisted on eliminating, as fast as possible, the lower levels, until the status of an institution of higher learning was at last achieved. All along the way he had had to fight the concessive spirit of the time. His faculty had complained that he "cut the sinews of their courage" when he had sent students on the preparatory school level to find their training in places especially designed to fit their needs.

In certain ways the development of the School of Nursing had been similar. Though high standards of admission were established at the start — of the thirty applicants who appeared in the first year the committee found only seven to have satisfactory qualifications — selection had to be based, in part, on the availability of candidates. The three-year program was designed to attract matriculants who did not expect to receive preparation leading to a degree. The nonexistence of any other kind of student made it necessary to admit the most promising ones to be found among young women who, in general, wanted vocational training.

But now the pioneer period was definitely over. Long since, the school had justified itself as a place where instruction could be offered on a high professional level. World War II had seen its rapid growth. Facilities had been improved by federal aid; a faculty of broad attainment had been brought together. The school was ready to do the work of a university, which is to prepare practitioners, teachers, and administrators in the broad functions of the profession.

Miss Densford and her faculty met with no such panic-stricken opposition as Folwell had had to face when they asked to drop the diploma program. During the spring of 1946 many groups were consulted — students, faculty, the advisory committee, the College of Medical Sciences. Of great significance to the future of the school was the support of the president of the university, James Lewis Morrill, who had been in office for just a year. Throughout these, and all later discussions, the prospects of the School of Nursing had the sympathetic attention of President Morrill. His philosophy that "education is indivisible" made ample room for the rights of nursing in a system of higher education. Any proposal that reached his desk for the advancement of the nurse's preparation had his immediate and thoughtful attention, and the school profited many times by his understanding and generosity. It had this kind of understanding in the major matter of redefining fundamental purpose.

The recommendation made by the faculty was that the school should admit both three-year and five-year students in the fall of 1946 but that in the spring of 1947 only candidates for the B.S. degree should be received. Loss of the diploma candidates would mean also a loss in enrollment. But no one felt that the sinews of his courage had been cut by the decision to do without them. In fact this action was in accord with the belief of the three-year graduates themselves. In answer to a questionnaire study, three fourths of them recommended that the school offer, on the undergraduate level, a baccalaureate program only.

It was true, also, that more and more incoming students wanted the degree program; for several years the number of other applicants had been steadily diminishing. There were enough diploma candidates whose training under the plan of the Cadet Corps had still to be completed; they would, of course, remain. Their company would cushion the drop in enrollment during the period of change. Another new group of students would be coming in under the terms of the GI bill of rights which offered free tuition to veterans of the services. Even without the three-year students the school was certain to have, when the anticipated bulge of enrollment in all university schools began to be experienced, numbers equal to those of pre-war days.

So, on July 12, 1946, the board of regents approved the recommendation of the Advisory Committee and a new phase of the school's history began.

Another impulse of reconversion was to consolidate gains made during the war in various fields of nursing service. One of these had to do with the care of patients in rural districts.

During the 1920's conscientious men like Dr. Mayo had been disturbed by the fact that the benefits of medical discovery often failed to reach people in scattered and isolated communities. These, in fact, had been tragically neglected. Since that time the state of Minnesota had seen great improvement in hospital care. Health insurance plans like that of Blue Cross were changing the outlook for care in rural cities and towns. Farm cooperative organizations had helped to establish many small hospitals of fifty, seventy-five, as many as a hundred beds.

A major problem still remained. Few nurses chose to go to these hospitals. The work of their wards was often conducted chiefly by attendants and aides. The rural hospitals needed better trained personnel.

In 1943 the School of Nursing had made a start toward developing among nurse students a great appreciation of the importance and interest of work in rural institutions. The experiment of sending students for active experience in small-town hospitals and in their communities was the first of its kind to be tried anywhere.

With the help of federal funds a demonstration project was conducted during twelve weeks of summer. On a volunteer basis fifteen seniors were sent in groups of three or four into the hospitals of towns having populations of 10,000 or less. The purposes were, first, to acquaint nurses who had been exposed only to conditions in big city institutions with the quite different environment of the rural hospital and of the surrounding community and, second, to persuade some of them that this was the sort of work to which they would like to give their lives.

These young women discovered that small hospitals were not necessarily makeshift affairs dependent on antiquated equipment and primitive techniques. Many were bright and comfortable places, modern in all respects of design and facility. Yet there were important dissimilarities of operation and of these the students made a thorough study.

Many aspects of learning were emphasized by the experience in rural nursing. One was the awareness that nursing should be practiced as a "family-centered procedure." This was always an essential item of the philosophy of the school and all its teaching. But in no other circumstance could it be so brilliantly highlighted. The nurse student traveled about the countryside with the county public health nurse. She visited the Farm Bureau, the county welfare office, the courthouse. She attended 4-H club meetings. Through these associations, many quite new to her, she became aware of the special health problems of the community. She saw the composite face of the family itself and recognized in its anxious look a tacit plea for attention to special needs.

The responsive young nurse began to understand the relationship of family background, occupation, isolation, economic status to the treatment of illness, physical or mental. She saw that a father's incapacity might mean the complete collapse of family economy through the loss of a crop; she saw that a mother's illness could mean the deflection and perhaps distortion of a child's way of life. And she saw all this more clearly than she had been able to do in a city institution the organization of which was based on a high degree of specialization. Her encounters with the rural physician showed that, though he was still the country doctor of a type thought to have been lost long since, he was quite astonishingly up-to-date in his knowledge of recent medical discoveries and of new techniques. At a moment's notice, one volunteer observed, he would travel far to care for "a new-born baby, grandpa's rheumatism or a sick bull." He would travel farther still to consult with specialists in the large cities about any difficult or unusual case.

The student was impressed also with the adaptability — and the sensitivity — of rural officials who would call a car and send X-ray machinery to a farmhouse rather than to require its sick occupant to report to the hospital.

Partly as a result of this experiment the faculty of the school began, in the mid-years of the 1940's, to explore other opportunities for giving students experience in the clinical specialties. A committee was assigned to the task of formulating a more complete general plan. Three of its members, Margaret Randall, Myrtle Kitchell, and Rena Boyle, drew up the first draft. Later rural nursing was fitted by Margery Low into the list of clinical specialties made available, as minors, to candidates for the B.S. degree.

Interest was now active in many quarters. A distinguished benefactor of education, the W. K. Kellogg Foundation, began offering appropriations to support experimental projects and Miss Densford applied for a share in these funds. The foundation had a nurse consultant on its staff (Mildred Tuttle then filled the assignment) and it took a particular interest in the work being done by the school in health protection.

At approximately the same time the Minnesota League of Nursing Education proposed that there be created a broad-scale program in rural nursing education which would be open to students in all schools of the state. Miss Densford was directly concerned with its development. So, too, was Rena Boyle who, as faculty member of the school and chairman of the League's curriculum committee, had a double interest. When the League formally asked Miss Densford to assume responsibility for the program in the entire state, she accepted despite the fact that once more her tasks were multiplied. This, she believed, was an obligation owed by a representative of a state university to the people of the state.

Three assets are required of an administrator in so large a project: wide experience in the actual practice of nursing, executive training, and ability to attract and hold the sympathetic cooperation of many different kinds of people. Katharine Densford possessed all of these to an unusual degree and her development of the state's rural nursing program stands as a major contribution to Minnesota's way of life. She was fortunate, also in having as chief deputy for the project a young woman of similar abilities. Margery Low (graduate in nursing, M.A., University of Minnesota) is a specialist in rural sociology and she brought many qualifications, both professional and personal, to the task.

So great was the success of the plan that, when the support which had been provided, first, by the Kellogg Foundation and, later, by Dr. Cowling, came to an end, something very like a public movement began to insure its continuation. Under the leadership of Mrs. Walter Walker a campaign of rescue work was launched. Like many another which has marked the history of Katharine Densford's contribution to public affairs, this one showed an effective pattern of faith supported by work. She and Mrs. Walker were able to obtain funds from many organizations and individuals to keep the program as an essential asset of community life. Beginning in 1956 the Minnesota legislature, recognizing the importance of the rural nursing project, has provided funds for support.

From the time in October, 1948, when the program had its modest beginning (there were just two students from two schools of nursing in two rural hospitals) it has grown steadily. Receiving hospitals, as of June, 1959, included the Lutheran Hospital, Bemidji; the Swift County–Benson Hospital, Benson; the Itasca Memorial Hospital, Grand Rapids; the Hibbing County Hospital, Hibbing; the Meeker County Memorial Hospital, Litchfield; the St. Michael's Hospital, Sauk Center; the Lakeview Memorial Hospital, Stillwater; the Northwestern Hospital, Thief River Falls; the Worthington Municipal Hospital, Worthington; and, functioning just in summer with students of the practical nursing programs, the Fairmont Community Hospital, Fairmont, and the Glencoe Municipal Hospital, Glencoe.

The enthusiasm represented by this broad participation reflects also the gratitude felt by the directors of all these Minnesota institutions for the benefits they have received. The experiment has affected the trend of nursing within the state. Beyond Minnesota's borders it has served as a pilot plan and helped many another institution to develop a similar plan.

A second large task of reconversion was that of unifying and expanding programs in psychiatric nursing. In this field, too, the war had stimulated special effort. The results of that effort, Miss Densford believed, must now be consolidated in a permanent plan of instruction.

During the years following the time when the progressive leadership of Dr. McKinley had resulted in the establishment at his university of a psychopathic unit for teaching and research, the neglect of disturbed patients had continued throughout the country as a whole. By 1940 the urgency of the situation had become generally apparent. As Walter Pitkin pointed out the number of cases of mental illness had multiplied, between the years 1880 and 1940, some twelve times over — "three times as fast as our wealth, four and a half times as fast as population, four times as fast as the number of school teachers."

The nursing committee of the American Psychiatric Association was deeply concerned about the poor prospects for the care of these sick minds because "the supply of adequately prepared nursing personnel appeared to be decreasing while the patient load was increasing." With funds from the Rockefeller Foundation the committee conducted a survey under the direction of nurse consultant Laura Wood Fitzsimmons. Her findings, published in 1943, showed that conditions were even worse than had been supposed. Private hospitals had one nurse for an average of sixteen patients, state hospitals an average of one nurse to four hundred patients. In one institution there was only one nurse for the whole psychiatric division and when she fell ill the patients were left with no professional care at all.

In 1944 a nationwide movement was launched to correct this appalling situation. Miss Densford, Dean Diehl, and Dr. Donald Church Balfour of the Mayo Clinic headed the Minnesota group. Because of the many contributions already made by the men of its psychopathic unit, the University of Minnesota was chosen by the American Psychiatric Association to conduct experiments in advanced training. By the end of the year three other such experiments were ready to be started at the Catholic University of America in Washington, D.C.; at the University of Washington in Seattle and at Ohio State University — all supported by funds from the Public Health Service.

Minnesota's program, begun in January, 1945, had as its head Mrs. Ione Slough, former superintendent of nurses at a public hospital in the state of Washington. She received active support from all the agencies associated in the project. A four-way partnership among the School of Nursing, the College of Medical Sciences, the Mayo Clinic, and the Rochester State Hospital provided the student with a unique experience. The contributions made by Dr. Balfour and Dr. Magnus C. Petersen, superintendent of the state hospital, combine to form a moving chapter in Minnesota's long history of cooperative enterprise in education.

Every phase of the program had the intense interest of a crucial experience. During their period of residence at Rochester nurse students worked directly with patients and at the same time took theoretical instruction from doctors of the Mayo Clinic. Dr. Balfour opened wide all facilities for study and, what is more remarkable, opened his own door — busy though he was in his triple role as teacher, investigator, and administrator — for frequent conferences. Dr. Francis Braceland met all students individually and interested himself to see that they had opportunity to study every kind of case. On the strictly academic side of the program experience was also rich. Dr. John Robson presented a brilliant course in neuroanatomy. Nurse students were encouraged to observe the work done in neurosurgery at the clinic and to follow postoperative care in particularly revealing cases.

At the end of the war Mrs. Slough resigned to go to Duke University. To succeed her Miss Densford fortunately secured an unusually well-trained teacher. Cecilia Lediger was the product of the war's furiously accelerated program in nursing education. She had earned her B.S. at Temple University and her M.A. at Teachers College, Columbia, when war caught her up. Assignment took her to the South Pacific where she served in a fatigue center established for the care of psychiatric cases. There she was under the guidance of an able director, Dr. Henry Davidson, who made sure that his nurses received deeply exploratory instruction. Her concern for this branch of nursing alerted by an exhausting but revealing experience, Miss Lediger went, after the conclusion of the war, to Mason General Hospital, Long Island, where she earned a special diploma in psychiatric nursing. When she joined the faculty of the Minnesota school of nursing, the entire country had just been shocked into awareness of the acute need for better psychiatric care.

PM was conducting a campaign to call attention to "The Shame of the Cities." Its articles exposed how grossly inadequate facilities were for the treatment, even for the shelter, of the mentally ill. As one case history revealed, a bedridden idiot had been refused admission to a state institution because of its "crowded condition." Year after year for three decades his parents asked repeatedly for help. Always it was denied while, in a series of bitter tragedies, father, mother, and sister sacrificed their lives to his care at home. To make the irony of this story completely unendurable it is necessary to add only, when the patient was at last received by an institution for the feebleminded, he died five days later.

It was evident that work of training nurses for this branch of their service must be speeded up — and not the day after tomorrow.

Many groups became active in the indirect service of nursing education as they campaigned for improvement in the care of the mentally ill. An organization of young Quakers took up the crusade. As conscientious objectors they had worked during the war as attendants in hospitals. Horrified by what they had seen, they joined with the National Committee for Mental Health to make a full report to the nation. The National Health Foundation, headed by Owen J. Roberts, earlier an associate justice of the Supreme Court, took up the cause with the eloquent support of such public figures as Pearl Buck, Dr. Harry Emerson Fosdick, Helen Hayes, William Green, and Sidney Hillman.

The time came presently when it appeared to organizers of this tremendous campaign of enlightenment that enough had been said about shame and that a word of hope might be spoken about the outlook for the future. The National Committee for Mental Hygiene prepared a group of radio scripts dramatizing the positive effects of care. The state hospital at Rochester, Minnesota, was chosen as a setting for the first of these, and the nurses of the university unit appeared in the documentary. The effect was all that could be wished. The general public had begun to lose its almost mystical fear of hearing mental illness discussed out loud.

A curative breath of fresh air was let into the atmosphere of the no man's land where the mental patients had existed so long. All through the centuries they had been regarded as children of disaster. (The word "child" was actually applied to any defective no matter what his age might be.) Now at last they were acknowledged by the general public to be the special protégés of science.

For this fortunate change in the lay mind the professional nurse deserves a large share of credit. Her work in helping to translate new theory into practice has done much to brush the cobweb of mystification and misunderstanding from traditional attitudes toward the mentally ill. A doctor could lecture for many hours on new approaches to treatment and care without achieving as much of a change in the average intelligence as is accomplished by the sight of a skillful nurse going cheerfully about a psychiatric ward treating sick people as though they are simply sick people with a good chance of getting well. It is her job to make a day-by-day and hour-by-hour routine of the altruism of science and she has learned it well.

The major result of the great campaign of the 40's on behalf of the mentally ill was the passage in 1947 of the National Mental Health bill which released funds for the training of personnel to put the new attitudes into general operation. But the University of Minnesota had not waited for this support for its own program. Again, through Mildred Tuttle, of the Kellogg Foundation, the School of Nursing had received the means of expanding its courses.

An influence was now at work in the minds of students which tended to make the short course of three quarters leading to a certificate in psychiatric nursing less attractive than one which existed as part of the Bachelor of Science program. The importance to the nurse of having the degree had been so widely stressed that more and more young women wanted to enter it while fewer applicants among graduate nurses applied for the certificate course.

During the late years of the 1940's Cecilia Lediger commuted between Rochester and the campus of the university directing two programs simultaneously. Emphasis had, of course, to be put on the program which students elected in greater numbers. Though it remained on the books of the school's schedule until 1950 the certificate program, with its practice center in Rochester, ended its effective history a year before. The loss of this unique project was regretted by everyone who had shared in it. But a university, being "a place where university work is done," must have its center where there are people to be prepared. And this, so far as psychiatric nursing is concerned, is now quite closely enclosed within the units on the campus. Again, the school had moved toward unity.

14

A Fresh Look at Nursing Needs

❧ THE promise that human life might be conducted once more on a basis of concern for normal interests, rather than of submission to the explosive demands of war, prompted Katharine Densford in 1946 to take what she called "a fresh look at nursing needs." It had been her undeflected determination even during the years of crisis to elevate the level of preparation for the nurse so that the superior product of a university school might, in turn, elevate the quality of patient care. This time of major readjustment to the practices of peace was the time also, she believed, for a broad extension of the outlook for her own field of education. Nursing is surely the oldest of the healing arts. But nothing would satisfy this tireless explorer of new possibilities but to see this art reborn, again and again, each time refreshed by an awareness of recent advances in science.

One thing of which Miss Densford and her faculty became sure, as they used their talents to make out the shape of the future, was that nurses returning to civilian duty after the war would want to investigate, more deeply than their original courses has enabled them to do, the work of the clinical specialties: medical nursing, pediatric nursing, psychiatric nursing, surgical nursing, obstetric nursing, operating room nursing. Crucial experiences of the war had aroused in the professional mind an active concern for the needs of all these areas of service. This interest must be captured and capitalized for the benefit of the whole tradition of health care. Questionnaires and surveys proved that a desire for new programs existed; the school felt an inescapable obligation to provide them.

This was the beginning of an ambitious new adventure in education which made a contribution of large importance to the history of nursing.

The first question to be decided was what place the graduate nurse student was to have in the scheme of academic life. This the faculty answered with the decision that she must be a student in the true sense. Like matriculants in any other college of the university system she was to pay tuition and fees and be responsible for her own maintenance. Plans of study were to be made for her on an individual basis so that her special interests might be fully satisfied. All graduate nurses who presented themselves for registration in the degree program were to be fully informed of the minor in clinical study which was now for the first time made available to them.

The second question was the ever-present one of how the new programs were to be supported. Miss Densford solved this with her usual persuasiveness by an appeal to the W. K. Kellogg Foundation. This generous friend of education agreed to grant funds at the rate of nearly $30,000 a year for a period of experimentation which in in the end covered five years.

Another absolute necessity was to find a director of this group of new offerings, for it was evident that much time would be required to explore possible fields of experience, to plan courses and to coordinate activities. Mrs. Coe, who had pioneered with the program of instruction for graduate nurses during the depression, was the obvious choice for this assignment and she accepted it. She had been active in university work of various kinds ever since her arrival in Minnesota. During Miss Densford's sabbatical leave in 1937-38 she had shared major teaching responsibilities in the School of Nursing with Lucile Petry. Later, Miss Densford's principle of encouraging teachers always to be learners had opened many opportunities to her to accept part-time assignments while she continued her studies. She had taken all the university's courses in pathology and, having found that she wanted to explore "the whys of functioning" deeper still, began an intensive program in physiology. In partnership with a young man, John Coe, whom she later married, she had begun work for a Ph.D. During the war years when many staff members had gone into military service she was virtually drafted to teach physiology and to assist in physiological chemistry.

Pressing and immediate responsibilities which were forever being presented to this extraordinarily useful woman prevented her from completing the one remaining requirement for the Ph.D. — a dissertation. But Mrs. Coe has had the compensatory satisfaction of being not merely a conspicuous innovator of new projects in nursing education but an inexhaustible public servant in such assignments as that of the vice-presidency of the American Nurses Association and active executive committee work for the American Heart Association and the earlier American Council of Rheumatic Fever.

The first two programs in advanced clinical nursing were developed in the areas of medical and pediatric care. Mrs. Coe herself assumed the teaching responsibilities in the first. To the second came a vivid product of the international tradition in nursing. Mrs. Ching-ho Liu Chu had been educated in a striking variety of schools all the way from Peiping, China, to Minneapolis, Minnesota. She was persuaded to interrupt her work for a doctoral degree at Columbia to help launch the new propect. Her high degree of preparation in the field of child psychology, as well as in the whole realm of child education and care, made her an unusually valuable acquisition even though she was able to remain for only a year.

Indeed, the news that a project of genuine significance had been inaugurated at Minnesota brought excellent teachers from everywhere. In the winter quarter Ruth Wiese was appointed to carry the responsibility for instruction in advanced operating room nursing and also in surgical nursing. In the second year of the undertaking Myrtle Brown replaced Mrs. Chu. Cecilia Lediger was brought into the program to expand activities in the psychiatric field. Alma Sparrow was appointed to the advanced clinical faculty to strengthen the social and community aspects of nursing in the advanced as well as in other curriculums. Katherine Kendall became responsible for advanced obstetric nursing. Each of these faculty members was already an expert in the clinical specialty for which she took responsibility at the time when she entered the school. The high level of preparation each had attained made her not merely an effective supporter of the program as a whole but an enthusiastic innovator of new enterprises in her own field.

In the five years of steady expansion made possible by the Kellogg grant, the project developed into an asset of the greatest importance to the entire community and was recognized as such by the hundreds of men and women who became concerned in its enterprises and eager to further its objectives. A company of extraordinarily able teachers continued in later phases to pour fresh energies into the ever growing program just as they did at the start. Helen Hanson entered the surgical area; Margery Low developed the interests of the plan in the field of rural nursing; Helen Bowditch and Helen Linehan joined the group of teachers in psychiatric work as did also Edith Mewhort, Lois Anderson, and Kathleen Black. (Miss Black later became director of the Mental Health and Psychiatric Nursing Advisory Service of the National League for Nursing.) In one moment of almost incredible expansiveness eight new members were added to the faculty.

As these programs go on today they benefit from the fact that in the beginning a clearly formulated philosophy guided the work of designing them. Fundamentally, of course, the purpose of the advanced clinical studies is to help students to "acquire knowledge and skills beyond those acquired during the basic nursing course." But enclosing this intent and supporting it on all sides are attitudes toward the responsibility of the nurse which teachers undertake to inculcate in their students. As "participating health-minded community citizens" nurses have a special duty to safeguard well-being as much as to care for sickness. They must be aware of the positive approach to the establishment of public health through teaching in the schools, beginning with that on the nursery level, and proceeding through that of all counseling offices in homes for the aged. They must be taught to understand the emotional and psychological aspects of health and disease in order to provide the pattern of nursing care needed by each particular patient. They must become well acquainted with the resources of their own community for care of illnesses of every kind so that their patients may share the benefit of their broad training. They must learn to plan with other health agencies for the continuing care of chronically sick patients. In short they must help to prevent disease if they can, "personalize" their nursing of patients when disease occurs, and plan for rehabilitation when the patient is on the mend.

To offer the nurse this kind of broad outlook on her profession Miss Densford and her faculty tirelessly canvassed the resources of their own community to find favorable areas of observation. These, they agreed, must be not merely in hospitals, clinics, health agencies, and public service organizations, but in business institutions as well. What they managed to create in the end was a vast laboratory of health and disease, the doors of which open on more than a hundred institutions and units of service where the problems of teaching people to stay well or of helping to shoulder their burdens of illness may be studied.

A catalogue of the agencies included in the work of the advanced clinical program may help to suggest its scope. In the field of operating-room nursing the facilities include many units of the university hospitals including operating rooms, outpatient department, radiotherapy department, the cancer detection center, and the Variety Club Heart hospital. In pediatrics, facilities include besides the university's own units of treatment and care many opportunities for observation in nursery schools, schools for exceptional children and places like the Gillette Hospital where the special responsibility is the care of crippled children and ones in need of orthopedic correction. In psychiatry the resources are particularly numerous, including every kind of service from the Minnesota Mental Health Society to the Rochester State Hospital and Alcoholics Anonymous. In surgery nothing is neglected — from the use of clinical facilities within the hospitals to tours of recovery rooms in other hospitals, visits to homes for the aged and even the offices of artificial limb companies.

In the course of this exhaustive tour of duty, health is presented to the nurse as an asset to be preserved by the power of education; it is presented as a value threatened, one which the subtle and scrupulous arts of scientific nursing must help to defend; it is presented as a value lost, yet one which must be offered the compensations which psychological understanding can supply. In this striking demonstration of how the cooperative temper can be put to work in the service of a common cause, the School of Nursing has presented evidence of its ability to unify and give direction to all the forces of education.

In 1951 when this project had established itself as an essential part of the nursing program in the estimation of all experts in the field, its existence was threatened. The Kellogg support came to an end, and the university was, at the moment, unable to assume financial responsibility. It was a dramatic moment for, as the end of one academic year approached and the opening of another loomed, both emptyhanded, beyond there seemed to be no hope for the program. Faculty members would have to find other assignments; the project would collapse; and the effectiveness of five years of effort would have been, in the end, for nothing.

In this crisis Miss Densford turned to Dr. Donald J. Cowling, then chairman of the Mayo Memorial Committee.

Dr. Cowling entered administrative work in 1909, the youngest president up to that time to take over the affairs of an important institution of higher learning. For thirty-six years thereafter he guided the destinies of Carleton College, at Northfield, Minnesota, leading it to distinction among cultural centers of its kind. When he retired in 1945 he did not propose to spend his leisure in contemplation of past achievements. Instead, he enlisted immediately in other educational causes. Several of these had to do with the plans of the University of Minnesota and some were concerned with proposals which, until Dr. Cowling adopted them, seemed entirely visionary. In each instance a unit of the university system had benefited in ways that will affect its future for generations to come.

What Miss Densford suggested to Dr. Cowling, when she approached him with the problem of how the advanced clinical programs might be continued, was characteristically modest. "I have come to you for advice," she said. Dr. Cowling listened to the story and his answer implied a characteristic decisiveness. "I shall not be of much use if I give you only advice."

Instead he went out and found the needed money — more than $50,000. The day was won; the life of the new program was assured for another two years without even a momentary pause in its progress.

As Dean Diehl once observed in recounting what he called Dr. Cowling's "heroic rescue": "It would have been nothing short of a calamity to discontinue this program at a time of such urgency."

The pleasant epilogue to the story came when another contest with the budget approached, and the state legislature was persuaded to accept Dean Diehl's view. The university itself was enabled by new appropriations to take over most of the program.

Another desire to adjust the traditional practices of instruction to the realities of modern society resulted in the establishment of a trial course in practical nursing. There are now more than five hundred such offerings in the schools of the United States, but the one started more than a decade ago at Minnesota has unusual features which give it special interest.

In 1946 Miss Densford pointed out that the greatly increased use of hospitals had made heavy demands on the nursing population. The need became apparent for a "group of carefully prepared people to assist the professional nurse." A committee of the school, headed by Thelma Dodds and including Ruth Harrington, Beatrice DeLue, and Agnes Love, drew up a plan for the creation of a program of instruction. Approved by the faculty of the school and by Dean Diehl, this program was authorized by the board of regents in 1947.

It is not difficult to imagine that the shades of many Minnesota men may have listened with interest in the background as these preliminary discussions went on. The lips of Dr. Mayo might have been seen shaping the words: "I always said there must a shorter program for nurses." Dean Lyon might have nodded approval for he had often pointed out that, as the nurse achieved the status almost of a "sub-doctor," other women must be recruited and prepared to work under guidance in performing the simpler tasks of daily routine. Even Dr. Beard's opposition would probably not have been implacable. The battle of standards has been won long since. The new proposal in no way threatened the prestige of the professional nurse.

Doubts that anyone may have entertained had to be balanced by other considerations. The University of Minnesota, as a land-grant college, is bound by many obligations to be "all things to all men." Over the years it has many times opened its doors to students who needed something other than highly specialized preparation in one or another of the professions or arts.

Into its School of Agriculture on the St. Paul campus it took — until its recent elimination from the Minnesota program — generation after generation of young people who wanted specific instruction in farm and home management. The General College, created in 1932, accepted the responsibility of meeting the needs of young men and women who do not expect to follow a full four-year course but want training to meet the problems of everyday life.

It has been the principle of the university when it makes such departure from academic tradition not to skimp the experiment at the start or to treat its interests with patronage. Over the development of the General College the president himself (the redoubtable Lotus Delta Coffman of the crusading 1930's) watched vigilantly, calling to his assistance many of his deans and many of his busiest, most distinguished research professors. General education, he believed, also has its standards and these must be kept high. With the persistence of the innovator he prodded every creative intelligence he could summon into offering ideas that would enable the program to endure and deserve to endure.

Similarly, Miss Densford insisted that the experiment in preparing practical nurses must represent no casual, no merely imitative, effort. Only the inauguration of a plan that would contribute something of permanent value to the profession could justify the attempt.

So the director of the school and her faculty entered with all conscientiousness into the task of making a new approach to the problem. Each of the two programs in practical nursing which its faculty designed had quite unusual features. These original developments were made possible by the fact that the university had, in the General College and the Institute of Agriculture, special facilities for the instruction of young people with particular needs.

A glance at the history of the practical nurse may serve to suggest why it became necessary to provide a definite formal preparation for her.

Before such a discipline existed, the term practical nurse had been used for many years to identify the untrained neighbor who came in to help during a family emergency. She was often a mature women with a family of her own. Sometimes she was a young girl who had always loved babies, a helper who could assume responsibility but who lacked training of any kind other than that derived from her native good sense.

As standards of health care rose throughout the country it became evident that preparation for assistants of this kind must be provided. Attempts were made as early as 1918 to establish centers of instruction. But these were sporadic and entirely inadequate to the need. It was only after World War II, when hospitals began to ask for more help than the nursing profession itself could supply, that a concentrated effort was made by leaders in the field to define what a practical nurse should be, to encourage programs for her education and to provide for licensure under state law.

Nursing organizations now agree that a practical nurse is
a person trained to care for selected convalescents, sub-acutely and chronically ill patients and to assist in the care of the more acutely ill. She provides nursing service in institutions and in private homes where she is prepared to give household assistance where necessary. She is employed by a private individual, a hospital or a health agency. A practi-

cal nurse works only under the direct orders of a licensed doctor or the supervision of a registered professional nurse.

The bulletin of the School of Nursing announced not one program but two: the Practical Nursing curriculum and the Practical Nursing and Home Management curriculum. The first was developed, from the beginning, with the participation of the General College. The second was offered in cooperation with the School of Agriculture.

The Practical Nursing curriculum covers four quarters of work done in residence on the Minneapolis campus. The faculty of the school serves all teaching functions; the university hospitals offer the major field of experience. Candidates for certificates must satisfy carefully regulated standards of admission. They must be at least seventeen years old. They must have high school diplomas or the equivalent, and they must take the pre-admission tests devised by the National League for Nursing. Marital status is not an admission consideration. The school wants students of good promise and it attempts to look only at the realities of potential contribution in making selections.

Instruction is liberal within the limits of the time allowed for preparation. Besides having clinical experience in the university hospitals the student in the practical nursing curriculum goes to the General College for courses in biology, psychology, social science, and nutrition. Indeed, the freest kind of interchange takes place between the two units. Many students who begin their post–high school careers in the General College later decide to enter the practical nursing program and many who begin in the practical nursing program decide to take their earned credits to the General College and work a second year for its degree, associate in arts.

One advantage gained by the school in having its own program for the preparation of practical nurses is that this provides a laboratory of human material in which a teacher-in-the-making may practice for her life work. A university school of nursing must send out, along with every other kind of instructor needed by the profession, ones who are prepared specifically to prepare, in their turn, the great company of practical nurses needed in hospitals and in the private care of patients. Teachers cannot practice effectively on any but actual pupils. Just as the University of Minnesota needs a nursery school and a high school in which the teachers of the future may encounter the actual conditions of their prospective jobs, so it needs to provide a controlled practice field for instructors of practical nursing. It is this aspect of the experiment which had decisive weight with the state legislature in persuading its members to endorse the plan and appropriate funds for its support. The effective preparation of those in whom the community must place its faith in education — that is to say, teachers on all levels and in every sort of relationship — has always been a consideration of chief importance in the minds of the men who make university appropriations.

The unique feature of the Minnesota plan is that it has been developed as a strictly educational program. Students assume the expense of their training, exactly as do students in other colleges, paying tuition fees, buying uniforms and textbooks. They do not receive maintenance in return for service given to the hospital during the training period. The advantage to both the student and the university is that classes and clinical experience can be arranged within the regular schoolday. Hospital practice is set up on the basis of the student's needs rather than on the basis of the needs of the hospital.

The second curriculum in practical nursing offered, while it was still in existence, an interesting example of how two units in a huge university system may work together, each adapting its special resources to the needs of the atypical student.

The purpose of the School of Agriculture was to give young people something more in the way of general education than they had had in their high school experiences. Ninety-five per cent of its students were high school graduates; the rest were people of mature years who were admitted on the basis of their individual abilities and classified as "adult specials." The program included courses in home management, household buying, and meal planning. It undertook, further, to throw light on matters that would concern these students later as citizens of small communities. They studied rural sanitation, rural sociology, aspects of American democracy, and art in everyday life.

For the greater part of the time that the school has been concerned with the problems of practical nursing the program has been in the hands of Eugenia Taylor. As the graduate of a three-year program Miss Taylor was acutely aware from the beginning of her career of the hospital's need of auxiliary personnel. Later studies for the B.S. and M.S. degrees at Minnesota have given her administrative experience and she brings to the development of practical nursing curriculums a double interest and a complete sympathy. Though her faculty, consisting of two members besides herself, never has been adequate to the size and scope of the programs, she has kept the offerings under constant review to the end that the experiment may produce effective results. She has consulted frequently with the faculties of the General College and of the Institute of Agriculture to improve offerings and to recruit the best possible candidates among students of the two branches.

The School of Nursing continues to regard the programs in practical nursing as experimental and all curriculums are to be reviewed for further appraisal of their place in a university system.

Meanwhile the undertaking has shown that the training of practical nurses can be conducted as a purely educational program; that the faculty of a university school can arrange a much more than ordinarily complete experience for workers of this kind; and that it can send such workers — mostly women — into the rural communities with a stimulated awareness of what their contribution to the work of health care can be.

15

No Ivory Towers

🌿 THE culminating achievement in the history of the School of Nursing during its first half century was the development of the advanced professional curriculums for which leaders had been pleading. To train high-level specialists, as well as the company of undergraduate students, is the proper work of a university school. Miss Densford and her faculty had moved steadily toward that goal despite all the difficulties that they encountered on the way. They had maneuvered themselves out of the blind alleys of budgetary limitation; they had fought their way through the exacting responsibilities and the formidable dislocations of war; they had won recognition and support from foundations and other outside sources of income to maintain original experiments in education. The end of an effort so thoughtful and so peristent should be the realization of a rich and varied system, covering the whole range of instruction. Fortunately, that realization has come about, as its bulletin testifies and as its reputation also testifies with emphatic approval.

Dr. Esther Lucile Brown, director of the Department of Studies for the Professions of the Russel Sage Foundation, has set forth what the objectives of the university school of nursing should be. They are first, "to prepare a group of nurses (estimated at some thirteen percent of the total number) who can fill administrative, supervisory, consultant teaching and research positions more nearly in conformity with current needs;" second, "to develop undergraduate curricula that attempt to lay a broader base in the physical, biological and social sciences;" third, "to seek systematically for urgently needed knowledge concerning patients' care and how such needs can be met."

To satisfy these needs in the fields of advanced study, undergraduate preparation and research, the School of Nursing at Minnesota undertook at the beginning of the decade a thorough revision and expansion of its offerings. The work of the decade produced, in the end, a general plan which one expert has called "the most complete, across-the-board program offered anywhere in the country today."

There are in this design three distinct curricula. The purpose of the first, the bachelor of science program in professional nursing, is "to prepare nurses for beginning positions in professional nursing under supervision in all areas." The purpose of the second — the programs in nursing education, one on the bachelor's, the other on the master's level — is to prepare professional nurses for positions which require an understanding of the principles and practices of instruction. The purpose of the third — the programs in nursing administration, of which, again, there are two, one on the bachelor's, the other on the master's level — is to prepare professional nurses for the work of directors and supervisors.

Some of these developed out of old programs; others were quite new; all were exhaustively studied, revised, and enriched during the period of creative activity in the 1950's.

Miss Densford and her faculty began their reconstruction work, at the foundation, with the basic professional program. To the class entering in September, 1949, the school offered for the first time a new four-year (sixteen-quarter) curriculum. This was not a streamlining of the old five-year plan but a reconceived pattern of instruction based on a new concept of responsibility toward the profession. In the eighteen-quarter curriculum of the past each student had, in addition to preparation for professional nursing, a major in nursing education or in public health nursing. The new plan shifts emphasis in order to give the student a broader background in general education. Her major is professional nursing and the focus of her concern during the years of clinical study is on patient care in its broadest aspects.

The program as a whole is designed to give the professional nurse, destined for general nursing duty, a lively awareness of the implications of her job as social service. It is based on the belief, once stated by Woodrow Wilson, that any profession is "clearly impoverished" which does not "draw to its special studies" men and women "bred to understand life and the broader relations of their profession."

The six quarters of prenursing instruction, which may be taken in any accredited college or university including, of course, the arts college of the university itself, are devoted to such studies as may be expected to alert the mind of the prospective student to appreciation of the relationship between a general subject and her particular duty. As one who must be able to communicate readily and confidently with patients she studies English and, for a further broadening of her sympathies, the humanities. As one who will presently be dealing with the complexities of adjustment either to mental patients or simply to the inevitable perturbations of illness, she must study psychology. As one who will have to do with sick children, she studies child development. As one who will learn that sickness affects and is affected by all human relations, she explores aspects of the social sciences — sociology, economics, or, if her tastes lead her in these directions, history and political science. As one who must soon advance to closer examinations of the basic sciences, she studies introductory chemistry and zoology. The day when the nursing student made her way through a "deadening routine" of chores, unlighted by any comprehension of the *whys* that lie behind the *hows* of her profession, is over for the matriculant in a modern school. No question could plague her in the daily round of the hospital to which she has not been offered some anticipatory guidance toward an answer.

Nurse students are encouraged to exercise wide choice among elective courses so that fundamental preferences may be stimulated and individuality of taste nourished. But their advisers in the School of Nursing keep scrutinizing eyes on their programs to make sure that a sense of direction is steadily maintained. The ninety-five quarter credits that must be earned in the prenursing schedule help to instil the "spirit of learning" which Wilson said must be the spirit of the technical laboratory.

During the ten quarters spent in residence in the School of Nursing and in clinical practice, the student follows a program of study similar to that which was established in earlier years but one that has been greatly deepened and broadened in content by the developments of modern science and by the fact that teaching methods have been steadily improved. She studies the biological sciences — elementary anatomy, general bacteriology, pharmacology, physiological chemistry, and human physiology. She pursues courses that have clear application to her needs in the School of Public Health and such studies as nutrition in the School of Home Economics. These are accompaniments of illuminating significance to work in the many phases of clinical nursing with which she is constantly occupied. Each of these activities is given added meaning by visits to observe the work of other agencies in some of which she has actual experience.

But it is the new emphasis on the individual and on an organized plan to give her a rich background of general education that gives the basic professional curriculum its distinctive character. Observers in other disciplines of the university system in whose classes nursing students take part testify that the plan has worked well. Because they have "grown up fast" in response to the well-defined promises of their future work, these young women are among the most responsive of their students.

The program is now the responsibility of Dorothy E. Titt, a widely experienced member of the school's faculty.

A major task to which Miss Densford and the faculty of the school addressed themselves after World War II was that of developing further what Lucile Petry Leone has called "the profession of teaching within the profession of nursing." As early as 1919 individual courses had been offered, in collaboration with the College of Education, that were designed to prepare teachers. These had already become well established and popular with students. But the profession's growing demand for instructors required that a university school should mine its resources of superior human material more thoroughly than ever to fill the large number of positions for which too few suitably trained applicants appeared.

Miss Densford brought to the problem her wide experience in making policy decisions for the profession. She had served as adviser to the army nurse corps in setting up educational programs for the services and in making concrete plans not merely for the immediate emergency but for the future. She had been an active worker on various committees of the National League of Nursing Education. She had been an alert and stimulating participant in many sessions of the International Council of Nurses, serving for several years as a vice-president. On all organizations of nurses within the state of Minnesota she had been an instigator of new enterprises. Co-workers testify enthusiastically that no president of the American Nurses' Association has ever presided over its huge sessions with so much authority blended with so much thoughtfulness and consideration. As Pearl McIver has said, the wonder among her associates ever grew that "one individual could keep her finger on so many graduate, undergraduate and practical nursing programs and in addition find time to think up new programs and new projects."

But new projects were precisely what interested Miss Densford most as she surveyed the outlook for nursing with keenly appraising eye. The loyalty that she inspired in her faculty and the resourcefulness that her example of foresighted planning aroused in its members enabled this cooperative group to share leadership in many kinds of advanced thinking for the profession.

To Ruth Harrington was delegated major responsibility for expanding the programs in nursing education more nearly to meet the requirements of the profession. Her colleagues, Rena Boyle and Sibyl Norris, became active and vigorous collaborators. Both had been Miss Harrington's students in the baccalaureate program and both were imbued with the spirit of the school's unwritten slogan: Anything can be tried at Minnesota; both were intimately acquainted with the educational resources of the community.

Rena Boyle had begun her work in nursing at Methodist Hospital, Peoria, and continued it at the University of Pittsburgh before coming to Minnesota. She had worked as a private duty nurse, an assignment for which she has a great respect as the one which makes the most important contribution to the welfare of the patient and to the help of the family in the crisis of illness. As teacher at Minnesota she had gained firsthand knowledge of the student mind and knew what attitudes, as well as what aptitudes, must be cultivated in those who undertake to instruct. Graduates of the programs at Minnesota remember with gratitude the staunchness of this adviser. Dr. Boyle's Junoesque stature and appearance, her imperturbable serenity of temper, the soundness of her instruction, and her sympathy in offering counsel all contribute to an image that remains for many that of the teacher with a true vocation.

Dr. Norris's enthusiasm for her job was of equal effectiveness. She herself remembers the fifteen years spent at Minnesota as a time when eagerness for new ventures and faith in young minds made confrontation of "the impossible" a pleasant feature of the daily routine. "Let us hear from some of the younger members," the director would say in faculty meetings. And: "Let us decide what we would like to do and worry about the money later." And in the end Miss Densford would announce: "The faculty decided what we must do."

Together these women worked out patterns of instruction in nursing education which would be expected to produce good teachers — ones who, in their turn, could train good nurses. The profession of teaching, they felt, had come of age and must now once more analyze its goals so that these might be clear to each instructor in classroom or clinical area. In the light of that analysis it seemed evident to them that emphasis must be shifted to a higher ground of educational method. It must move beyond the effort simply to prod or cajole students into mastering texts and memorizing steps in procedures, to the end that they might be able to pass examinations. Rather the teacher must learn to inspire in her students a desire to develop skill in solving patients' problems and to find deep satisfaction, as an individual worker, in bringing patients back to health, to security, to full functioning once more as human beings.

The first of the two programs in nursing education, that on the bachelor's level, is "designed," as the bulletin says, "to prepare professional nurses for head nurse, clinical supervisor and teaching positions in hospitals, clinics, health services and schools of professional and practical nursing and for other positions in which an understanding of educational principles and practices is needed."

The second program, leading to the degree of master of education in nursing education, has as its purpose preparing professional nurses "for positions in educational programs in nursing — basic professional schools, graduate nurse clinical programs and practical nursing programs — through a broad program of study and experience based upon undergraduate study and experience in nursing education."

In short, the object of the baccalaureate program is to produce teachers to fill jobs on a first level of responsibility, that of the master's program to produce teachers to fill jobs on a higher level of responsibility.

The typical candidate for the B.S. degree in nursing education enters with a diploma from an accredited school of nursing. Her home may have been in the Midwest, the east coast, the Pacific coast, or some foreign country. She travels far — or less far — seeking the varied experience that a recognized center of medical study has to offer. She must meet the entrance standards of the College of Education and those of the School of Nursing Admissions committee. For work done previously she receives blanket credits, a total of some 45 out of the 186 she must earn for her degree. She enters the university as a sophomore but, in her first year, takes the freshman subjects — English, sociology, general psychology, child psychology. She is encouraged to invite her soul in the choice of electives. That she does so with imagination and boldness is witnessed by the fact that nurse students have taken everything from music to instruction in flying.

The emphasis of the second year is on nursing. The student starts work on her minor in a clinical field which particularly attracts her. Each of these has its specific prerequisites which she must satisfy. In addition to these courses she takes electives plus other required courses in nursing among which are ward administration, personnel work, trends in nursing.

During her senior year the student is concerned chiefly with her major, education. The electives offered her have also direct reference to the job of becoming a good teacher and many take the popular course, Personality Development. But her preoccupying task is to study the principles of teaching both in theory and in practice. The College of Education collaborates closely with the school and in at least two of their courses nurse students study other areas of education than their own specific field. But the course Introduction to Teaching has been designed by faculty members of the School of Nursing to show the direct application of general method to the particular problems of instruction in the clinical situation.

The significant feature of the program is, of course, that it puts the student actively to work as a teacher. During her final academic year, under close supervision, she gains actual experience in teaching by serving in a school of the Twin Cities which collaborates with the university in this cooperative enterprise. In earlier years Dr. Boyle and Dr. Norris explored possibilities with persuasive enthusiasm and the school brought as many as seventeen outside institutions into the system.

Besides the strenuous labor of organization they found little difficulty in eliciting help. It would seem to be characteristic of the nursing profession that its members welcome new responsibilities if these show a direct relationship to the problem of improving patient care. Staffs of schools, hospitals, and other agencies in Minneapolis and St. Paul work with faculty and students of the university school generously and without financial remuneration. They do so in the belief that they help, first, to improve the service of their own institutions; second, to recruit promising teachers to their field; third, to elevate and standardize methods of instruction. But the encompassing consideration would still seem to be that they enjoy the work. In many a quietly dramatic session of the past Dr. Boyle and Dr. Norris watched anxiously for the response to suggestions for further expansion of the teacher training program only to find that directors of hospitals were running briskly at their right hands, ready and eager to catch up new tasks.

The advisers are responsible for the assignment of each student in nursing education to a particular school. A conscientious effort is made to suit individuality to individuality so that sympathy of outlook between the two may be as great as possible. Further, the student may be deliberately placed in a setting unlike what she has known before so that her experience may be broadened.

Students are observed daily in their classroom performance. Each of the present advisers in the baccalaureate program, Ruth Wiese and Frances Dunning, spends from thirty to thirty-five hours a week traveling from school to school, inspecting the work of practice teachers. This time-consuming procedure has many rewards, the chief of which is that it wakens a high degree of sensibility in both student and observer. The student-teacher does not work in the dark, unable to appraise her own effort. Her first class may be an ordeal, causing only panic as she sees notes being taken on her performance. But, in usual circumstances, all later classes are conducted in an atmosphere of absorbed calm, for the young practice teacher has learned that her mentors will apply the techniques of appraisal always with the positive purpose of improving method. The intention is, as Lucile Petry Leone has said, "to add richness and effectiveness to the student's analysis of problems."

The program has been popular, and its success may be measured by the fact that, as of August, 1958, it had returned to the "profession within the profession" some 675 well-prepared teachers.

The program for the master's degree in nursing education, offered for the first time by the School of Nursing at Minnesota in 1950, is similar in broad outline to that of the bachelor's program. There are, however, major differences in organization and others having to do with both the depth and breadth of study. Of more mature and more advanced students greater exactions are made exactly as they are made in any other college of the university system.

179

Candidates for the master's degree are registered in the College of Education. It has always been a point of pride at Minnesota that no walls have been allowed to be reared up around its units; no guards stand at the barriers to inspect academic visas. Collaboration between the College of Education and the School of Nursing has ever been intimate and such of its figures as the late dean, Wesley Peik, Dr. Marcia Edwards, Dr. Ruth Eckert, and Dr. C. Gilbert Wrenn offer examples of the skill with which men and women in one discipline can lend assistance to those in another. At commencement, graduates of the master's program in nursing education receive their awards at the hand of the dean of the College of Education though the major part of their work has been done in the School of Nursing.

During the quarter devoted to field experience, candidates for the master's degree act as associate teachers and participate fully in the concerns of the faculty in the cooperating institutions to which they are assigned. They help in the revision of the curriculum, attend appropriate committee meetings, and go as observers to professional conferences and association meetings. The major adviser follows the progress of each student at work in the school of assignment. On one day of each week candidates return to the campus for a seminar conducted by Miss Harrington to which they bring particular problems of teaching and supervision. These are submitted to discussion by the whole group.

The chief differences between the field experience in the bachelor's program and that in the master's program are, as the major adviser has stated them, "in scope and type of supervision." In the bachelor's program "the teaching experiences focus upon the guidance of learning in classroom and laboratory. Variety in the use of teaching method is sought; each class is carefully planned and supervised both as to content and method." The candidate for the master's degree is expected, because of her greater degree of experience and maturity, to be more nearly "self-directing." Though she, too, is responsible for "guidance of learning of individual students and groups of students," her responsibility as associate faculty member is much broader. Her self-dependent exploration of her field is guided by the "evaluation conference" in which major matters of teaching method are considered.

To fix attention productively on the daily task of patient care, each candidate for the master's degree is required to make a special study of some particular aspect of teaching, supervision, or management. Many of these have proved to be of immediate value to the cooperating agencies in the redesign of their programs and policies. The file of these investigations, kept in the office of the major adviser, constitutes a pool of information such as Florence Nightingale urged the profession to establish. It might well be explored by research workers of the future to assist the advance of teaching method and of curriculum management.

The development of the third curriculum, nursing service administration, very particularly concerned Miss Densford and the faculty of the school during the 1950's. Indeed, it demanded concentrated effort of all the leading university schools of the country.

The dean of one of these schools made the statement in 1957 that "Six years ago nursing service administration was almost an unknown term in the vocabulary of nursing. Now, the development of leaders for hospital nursing services is receiving as great, if not greater, attention than any other phase of nursing education."

There were many reasons for this sharp awareness of need. World War II had stimulated brilliant advances in medical science. Americans throughout the country wanted to profit by these improvements in treatment. The demand for hospital service increased. As a result of this demand many new hospitals were built and old ones enlarged. The outlook for the success of previously unimagined surgical operations brightened dramatically and patients filled the new hospitals. Prepayment plans for medical expense put the benefits of all these advances within the reach of the many.

An inevitable result of this wide demand for care was that the work of the hospital became much heavier and infinitely more complex. Because of the shortage of nurses during the war, a corps of auxiliary assistants had been brought in and their number steadily increased. These men and women — practical nurses, nurses' aides, orderlies, and ward clerks — required supervision. But there were far too few of such supervisors to meet the demand and even those who were engaged in administrative work felt themselves to have been insufficiently prepared for their assignments. In short, a new kind of nursing responsibility had developed out of new conditions. The profession was agreed that educational programs in nursing administration must be offered by the university schools and that these must come into existence quickly.

For many years the School of Nursing at Minnesota had offered individual courses in such subjects as hospital economics and ward administration. Its own view of the imperative need for broader instruction was that two goals must be accomplished simultaneously: first, adequate preparation must be provided for directors, assistant directors, and supervisors of the many-sided operation that nursing service had become; second, improvement must be made in the laboratory areas used for the education of nurse students.

In response to requests from the University of Minnesota School of Nursing and other collegiate schools, the W. K. Kellogg Foundation agreed, in 1950, to provide funds for an exploratory study of nursing service administration. Under the direction of Herman S. Finer (D.Sc., professor of political science, University of Chicago) a seminar of nurse administrators and nurse educators examined various aspects of the problem from January 15 through June 8, 1950. Minnesota's representatives at the Chicago seminar were Thelma Dodds, director of nursing at the Miller Hospital (a participating agency of the university) and Florence Julian, then assistant director (now director) of nursing services in its own hospitals.

Following this session plans were formulated for the Master of Nursing Administration program. Its design adapted recommendations of the seminar report to the facilities and resources of the Minnesota school. In the fall of 1951 Helen Goodale (Florentine) assumed major responsibility for the program and the first four students were admitted. A five-year grant from the Kellogg Foundation assured support during the developmental stages of the new offering in higher education for the nurse. The agreement contained the understanding that the University of Minnesota would gradually assume financial responsibility for its continuance. Margaret Grainger (A.B., Butler University, M.S., Teachers College, Columbia) taught and guided field experience in ward administration, a sequence which had been instituted earlier by Margaret Randall (Van Alystine). The coordination of well-established activities with ones that were quite new produced the curriculum of the master's program.

Its emphases, all developed on a basis of individual consultation between a candidate and her adviser, are quite clear. Three phases of the program stress, first, principles of administration applied to nursing service; second, the broader aspects of administrative problems; and third, original investigative study. To satisfy requirements in the first of

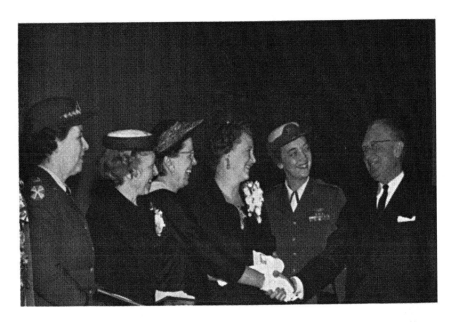

Recipients of the University's Distinguished Achievement Award: top, Inez Haynes, Mildred L. Montag, Myrtle Kitchell Aydelotte, Rena E. Boyle, Frances I. Lay, (James L. Morrill); bottom, Dorothy Kurtzman, Cecilia Hauge, Agnes Love, Anna J. Mariette, Barbara Thompson Sharpless

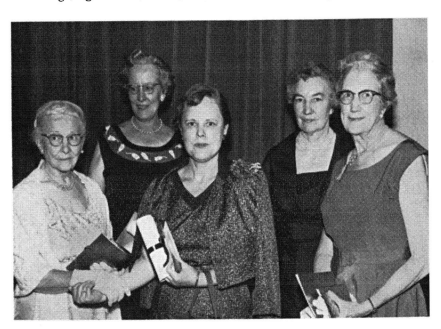

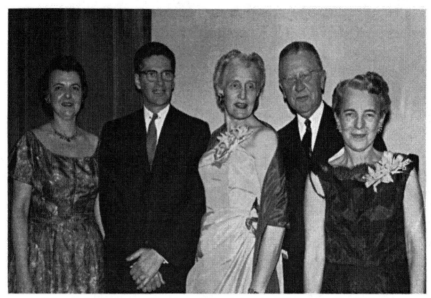

Edna Fritz, present director of the School of Nursing, Dr. Robert
B. Howard, dean of the Medical School, Katharine Densford,
President Morrill, Lucile Petry Leone

The fiftieth-anniversary banquet

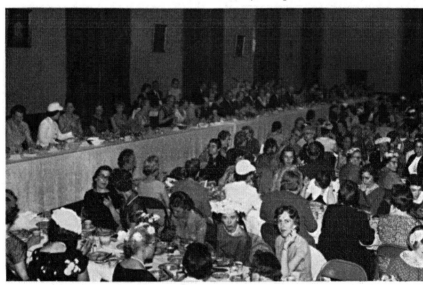

these subdivisions of interest the candidate at Minnesota takes a sequence of nursing service administrative courses developed by the faculty of the school and taught in its own classrooms. To give her the liveliest possible awareness of responsibility in the field of human relations, she reports to various units of the university system for different kinds of professional instruction. She goes to the School of Public Health to take a required course in the history and development of hospitals. In the department of political science she studies a course, also required, in municipal administration or one in public administration. The School of Business Administration provides still another required course in principles of industrial relations. Other electives are available, all having direct relationship of one sort or another to her special interest. Finally, to gain actual administrative experience, she has field practice in one of the cooperating hospitals which may be in the Twin Cities or in a smaller community of the region. During this period she acts as deputy to the director of nursing service, participates in the full range of her activities, and plans and conducts a project of her own — that is, a systematic study of a selected administrative problem.

Two additional objectives were included in the inclusive plan for development in the field of nursing administration. One was "to give as much assistance as possible to employed nurses in Minnesota, and throughout neighboring states, by offering extension courses, institutes, workshops and consultation services." The second was "to enrich the nursing administration content in the program of basic students through curriculum study, consultation with faculty members in the basic curriculum and participation in the teaching program for basic students."

While the master's program was being developed faculty members of the School of Nursing became more and more acutely aware of another need in the field of nursing service administration. M.A.'s in nursing from the Minnesota school have been called upon for many years to serve a region that reaches beyond the limits of the state. No program comparable to that of the master's plan at Minnesota is available to nurses living in Wisconsin, North Dakota, or South Dakota. This North Central region of the United States is predominantly rural; many small hospitals serve the scattered population. The need for nurses to fill administrative positions is large. Executives of the rural hospitals had to meet it, in the early years of the 1950's, by appointing to such jobs nurses who in a majority of instances were graduates of three-year programs. The percentage among them of nurses holding baccalaureate degrees was small.

To the faculty of the Minnesota school it seemed probable that many of the small hospitals could not look forward to a time in the near future when they would be able to afford even one nursing administrator prepared at the master's level. However, the administrative problems of the small rural hospital are no less difficult and pressing than those of larger, more affluent hospitals. The faculty, therefore, felt a responsibility to improve the nursing care of patients by preparing another sizable company of nurses to enter this kind of service.

A new program for full-time students was required. Extension courses were helpful but broader preparation was needed and was frequently requested by many nurses. What they wanted was an education that would fit them to become team leaders, head nurses, and supervisors. In such posts they could, of course, serve in urban as well as in rural hospitals.

With these needs in mind Miss Densford and the faculty of the school developed the baccalaureate program with a major in nursing service administration. Participants in its design were the originators of the master's plan with Isabel Harris, Myrtle Kitchell (Aydelotte), Florence Brennan, and Doris Miller added.

The baccalaureate program in nursing administration established in 1954 has grown steadily in enrollment. The first class, graduated in 1956, had nine members; that of the year 1956–57, thirty-nine. The strength of the year which marked its fifth anniversary was forty-six.

One way in which both the master's and the baccalaureate programs in nursing administration have been particularly fortunate has to do with the development of field experience. Faculty members of the Minnesota school feel that those with whom they cooperate in hospitals of the region have responded with the liveliest kind of sympathy in providing opportunities for students to observe and participate in active and effective nursing activities. Personnel of the various agencies have expressed, quite spontaneously, the feeling that they receive stimulation from the presence of students among them. For their part, university faculty members benefit from close association with practitioners and from intimate identification with their problems as well as with their achievements.

Besides the director of the school and Miss Harrington, who is in general charge of all the school's programs in higher education, major advisers of the curriculums in nursing administration now are Isabel Harris, Margaret Grainger, and Hannah Walseth. Miss Harris, who has earned degrees on successive academic levels from the University of Michigan, Johns Hopkins School of Nursing, and the University of Minnesota, has had wide experience in nursing (her army service included four years in the South Pacific) teaching, supervising, planning of curriculums, and administrative work. She is now lecturer and assistant to the director of the school. Miss Grainger is an expert in several fields of administration, most particularly that of team nursing. She is in constant demand throughout the Upper Midwest region as consultant, conductor of workshops, and lecturer. Miss Walseth is a representative of the generation of students who have been reared in the new tradition of nursing service administration; she approaches the problems of its further development with a belief in its purposes which supports and will help to fulfill the belief of her colleagues.

The competent strides by which Miss Densford and her faculty made their way during the 1950's toward the fullest possible program for the higher education of the nurse covered a significant distance between old ways and new. They have helped to conquer new ground for the profession. The respect with which the advanced curriculums are regarded by the whole university community emphasizes the general belief that the school has established a solid position for nursing education as an essential part of the work of a genuine university. The master's programs crown all other accomplishments of the period. The world of educators is in complete agreement that these are no ivory towers to which the nurse retires to gratify a taste for contemplation. They are centers for study of the immediate realities of human need and for the improvement of service to meet those needs. They are essential to the profession, surely; far more than that they have demonstrated in successes of many kinds that they are essential to the well-being of humankind.

16

The University, the Colleges, and the School

IN NOVEMBER, 1909, at the moment when the first university school of nursing had just made its debut, there appeared in the *Delineator* magazine an article by Woodrow Wilson, then president of Princeton University, which set forth his "Ideal for the True University." Wilson's central point was that in the emergent philosophy of American education, stress must be laid on the desirability of having the professional schools — law, medicine, engineering, and the rest — closely integrated in a university system of which a liberal arts college was the foundation.

Technical schools would find — so ran Wilson's argument — that "their practical, definite utilitarian objects" were fulfilled best in a university where many different interests cooperated to work "the fertile soil of catholic knowledge and inquiry." Students of a particular discipline should be "first of all citizens of the intellectual and social world — first of all university men with a broad outlook on the various knowledge of the world and *then* experts in a great practical profession." The colleges and schools of a university should be "vitally united from end to end." The permanent ideal for the American system of education should be that of serving "the intellectual needs of the age, not in one thing, not in one way only, but all around the circle with a various and universal adaptation to their age and generation."

Wilson's was, perhaps, the most complete and explicit expression, made up to that time, of a belief which was guiding the development of the large state universities. The same principle was enunciated many times over by each in turn of Minnesota's leading educators. The first president of the university, Folwell, had had a clear concept of what

186

he called the "genuine university," equipped to train men and women each for a special kind of public service but qualified also to awaken a vivid awareness of the whole range of social responsibility. Northrop had concentrated during his long administration on recommending the university system to any who might continue to be dubious about its ability to provide a liberal education which should be also an education in ethics; this service, much needed at the moment, he performed admirably. Again, Vincent's concern was with the system as a whole. He poured new blood into each unit; these transfusions of scholarship were given to medical school, law school, arts college, college of education so that all might contribute to the health of the institution. Coffman, facing the formidable trials of the 1920's and 1930's, played no favorites as he urged each unit on toward distinction; as he once said bluntly he intended to allow no particular college of the system to become "the tail that wagged the dog." Guy Stanton Ford, who had been dean of the graduate school for many years before becoming president of the university, had a broad knowledge of the resources of the educational world and he explored that acquaintance wisely to bring in men who could improve both teaching and research activities, quite as much in medicine as in the arts college, quite as much in agriculture as in any other unit of instruction.

In a memorable episode of his career as administrator, Walter Coffey dramatized this philosophy of oneness. When he came to Minnesota as dean of the agricultural college, a group of well-meaning members of the farming community entertained him at luncheon and in the course of the hospitalities a spokesman for the group made an unguarded comment. "We want you to know," he said in effect, "that we don't care what becomes of the rest of the university but that you can have anything you want." Coffey thanked his hosts for their vote of confidence but added soberly: "I must tell you that I could accept nothing for my own college that would not be for the good of the university as a whole." When later he moved into the president's chair during the years of World War II the same philosophy governed each of his decisions.

In recent years the idea has been more clearly stressed than ever before. President Morrill's belief that "education is indivisible" assured the rights of each unit, for he regarded each not merely as an integral but as an organic part of the whole.

These attitudes of mutual respect and mutual dependence have created at Minnesota an atmosphere in which the faculties of all branches take satisfaction. They believed that an equable climate of cooperation has warmed and encouraged growth in usefulness.

From its earliest days the School of Nursing had close links with many colleges on the campus. Student nurses received instruction in classes of the arts college, the college of education, various departments of the college of engineering, and the department of public health. Its most intimate association of all was inevitably with the medical school which, to begin with, supplied a good measure of instruction, especially in science courses.

The cooperation between the School of Nursing and the medical school begins with the preparation of the year's work. The director of the one informs the dean of the other in what departments her students will need instruction; the dean passes on to heads of faculties responsibility for supplying it. Dean Lyon's strong conviction about the importance of training the nurse in the fundamental sciences assured to the director the most sincere and sympathetic help. Opportunities of preparation for the nurse must be broad and searching, Lyon told his colleagues. His policy is followed today by all department heads and instructors in the College of Medical Sciences to whom the director or faculty representative of the school now makes requests directly.

It has been an enormous advantage to the School of Nursing that it exists in a place where every kind of educational experience is available and where the particular concerns of the profession are fostered in a college of medical sciences which has grown steadily in distinction.

A striking figure of an earlier period in the development of a design for instruction in nursing at Minnesota was Dr. Esther M. Greisheimer. In the company of those who "gladly teach" she was long conspicuous not merely for devotion to her job but for the skill with which she opened up the intricacies of rapidly growing knowledge in the fields of physiology and physiological chemistry. Broadly trained in her specialty (B.S., Ohio University; Ph.D., University of Chicago; M.D., University of Minnesota), Dr. Greisheimer prepared a large number of men and women who occupy important places in the world of science today throughout the country. The dedication of her frequently reprinted textbook, *Anatomy and Physiology*, to Katharine Densford and to the groups of nurses "whom it has been my joy to teach" indicates the particular emphasis which in the past Dr. Greisheimer, now professor at Temple University, Philadelphia, has placed on the preparation of women for a vital profession. Her example stands, along with that of such men as L. Earle Arnow (now president of the Warner Lambert Research Institute), bearing witness to the earnestness with which scholars at Minnesota have dedicated their efforts to the task of providing the nurse with a truly liberal education.

Today, many men carry on the tradition. Among them are the heads of departments in the College of Medical Sciences; the Doctors Arnold Lazarow in anatomy; Frederick H. Van Bergen in anesthesiology; Jerome T. Syverton in bacteriology and immunology; Cecil J. Watson in medicine; John L. McKelvey in obstetrics and gynecology; John E. Harris in ophthalmology; Lawrence R. Boies in otolaryngology; John A. Anderson in pediatrics; Raymond N. Bieter in pharmacology; Frederic J. Kottke in physical medicine and rehabilitation; Maurice B. Visscher in physiology; Wallace D. Armstrong in physiological chemistry; Donald W. Hastings in psychiatry and neurology; Gaylord W. Anderson in public health; Harold O. Peterson in radiology; and Owen H. Wangensteen in surgery. Also the directors of divisions: the Doctors Francis W. Lynch in dermatology; Gerald T. Evans in clinical laboratory medicine; Starke R. Hathaway in clinical psychology; A. B. Baker in neurology; William C. Bernstein in proctology; William T. Peyton in neurosurgery; John H. Moe in orthopedic surgery; and Charles Creevy in neurology.

Ray Amberg, administrator of hospitals, has worked closely with the director of the school as did his predecessors before him — Dr. Baldwin, Mr. Paul Fesler, and Dr. Halbert Dunn. Through many changes of policy with regard to such matters as the number of hours to which students were assigned for experience in the various departments, the final effect of this collaboration has been, in each phase, a steady improvement in the quality of clinical teaching.

It is a further advantage to the nurse student at Minnesota that she makes her way toward a full understanding of the complexities of her job in an atmosphere that is illuminated by hope for the future. Her studies are conducted in a place where the care of the patient is always the first consideration but where a second concern is ever present in the minds of a great majority of the medical men with whom she is associated. This is the obligation of the investigator to try to make some permanent contribution to the welfare of humanity through the conquest of disease. Scores of researches are being conducted today, and to all clinical work involved in many of these studies the nurse makes a significant contribution.

In the year 1950, Dr. E. T. Bell, looking back with the detached and impersonal eye of a retired professor, surveyed the history of the medical school on the faculty of which he himself had served with long and conspicuous success.

During the past two score years the Medical School has developed from a second class teaching unit to one of the foremost research institutions in the country. [How has] this remarkable change been brought about? The strength of a medical school is proportionate to the number of recognized leaders of medical thought on its faculty. Good teaching is necessary and not incompatible with investigation; but only research men make a university famous. The primary purpose of a medical school is to train young men and women; but it has also the obligation to advance medical knowledge. A department that does not encourage investigative work soon stagnates and even its teaching deteriorates. [At Minnesota] from 1913 onward there has been continuous progress in most departments due to the appointment and promotion of outstanding men.

The entire Minnesota community is proudly aware of the contribution now being made by the faculty in the College of Medical Sciences to the research programs of the United States. The nurse is still more proud, because she is far more intimately aware, of these significant achievements. She follows and administers the innovations in cancer treatment that have resulted from the investigations of a closely collaborating team of scholars working in the many divisions. In recent years she has participated, at the sides of their originators, in the development of new techniques in surgery: gastric resection operations, new treatments of postoperative conditions, development of cross-circulation methods, the dramatic success of "open heart" surgery — all these have won international recognition. No less important than these unique and spectacular advances which have brought observers from all over the world is the very impressive program of patient day-by-day exploration into many fields. At Minnesota important advances have been made in the study of polio, hepatitis, rheumatic fever, brucellosis, the virus diseases, epilepsy. The college's research men have achieved original contributions in the study of intestinal obstruction and kidney disease. To the nurse student the names associated with all these studies, innovations, and discoveries are not mere glittering symbols of the spirit of science; they are attached firmly to men whom she knows and with whom she works: the Doctors Wangensteen, Watson, Visscher, Armstrong, Bittner, Spink, Lillehei, Varco, DeWall, Wannamaker, Good, and many others. Daily she breathes the invigorating air of a place where experimentation is a matter of routine and where discovery often brings — to her as well as to investigators — the quiet elation of knowing that a problem has been met, a difficulty surmounted.

It would be surprising if such an atmosphere were not stimulating and Lucile Petry Leone has testified from personal recollection of her days at Minnesota that students have, in fact, always responded to it.

The focus of the university hospitals was always on patient care. What student nurses learned from their brilliant teachers they were eager, each as an individual and all as members of a team, to carry to patients. The benefits of modern science, received so directly from their originators, were to students no bits of abstract instruction but immediate realities to be used to ease suffering and to transmit hope.

From the days of incredibly meager beginnings when internes carried patients on their backs from bed up a narrow flight of stairs to the operating room, the facilities of the place in which the nurse student follows the round of care and learns her job have improved until they have become equal to any that exist in the modern world. Undergraduate and master's candidates benefit alike, in the quality of their preparation, by the fact that their setting is an important medical center.

Many factors have contributed to the growth of this institution. One is that the College of Medical Sciences has attracted generous support not merely from the legislature but from private individuals and from public figures who have recognized the importance of unifying, improving, and expanding the means of educating students in medicine.

First of the steps forward, in point of time, was the establishment, in 1915, of the Mayo Foundation. With a striking display of public spirit, the brothers Mayo, heads of the famous clinic at Rochester, Minnesota, decided that a share in the rewards that had come to them "from the people" belonged "to the people." They offered to make return in the form of an endowment for an unusual teaching unit. This placed the entire facilities of the Mayo Clinic within the graduate medical teaching program of the university. During their lifetimes Dr. Charles and Dr. Will Mayo, acting as private persons, gave some three million dollars to the foundation. Its existence has greatly extended opportunities for training physicians. It has helped also to improve opportunities for nurses who, in their advanced clinical studies, encountered at the Mayo Clinic a second distinguished faculty and had their area of field experience broadened far beyond the limits of the ordinary training program.

During the decade of the 1920's a succession of private benefactors, inspired, in part, by the example of the Doctors Mayo, came forward with gifts to the university for improvement of its hospital facilities. With the addition in 1924 of the Todd Eye, Ear, Nose and Throat Hospital and of the George Chase Christian Memorial Hospital and Institute it became necessary to speak, not of the university hospital, but of the university hospitals. The Eustis Children's Hospital and the University Hospitals Outpatient Department — both constructed in 1929 — added to an ambitious program of service. In each of these units, too, the student nurse found unusual opportunities to study the care of patients. Because each was dedicated to the investigation of the causes of disease, as well as to its treatment, work in the hospitals was conducted constantly under the revealing light of a concern for the fundamental principles of improving the human condition.

A later addition to the group of institutions within the university's health center is the Variety Club Heart Hospital, completed in 1951. This unit offers another dramatic example of altruism at work. Almost twenty years ago an organization of theater men of the region decided that it must be their contribution to the public cause to help the university study heart conditions in children who have suffered from rheumatic fever. How this particular inspiration happened to come to them is unimportant as compared with the moving fact that the benevolent obsession grew and grew in the minds of the showmen until their efforts had managed to create another important unit in the university's research system. As President Morrill has said, the Heart Hospital as it exists today "is splendid with vivid colors and flooded with daylight — in harmony with the bright promise it holds for those who come there under a cloud." It is devoted, in part, to infectious diseases of the heart and, in part, to the study of degenerative types of cardiovascular disease such as coronary occlusion, arteriosclerosis, and hypertension. In it, the nurse along with the medical student has another rare opportunity to study at an important center of exploratory investigation, the latest methods of treatment and care.

The most dramatic adventure of all, in the history of the development of a huge medical center at the University of Minnesota, was brought to fulfillment with the dedication on October 21, 1954, of the Mayo Memorial. This building towers fourteen stories high, above the cluster of older medical units. As a symbol it encloses in the solidity of brick and mortar the respect which the people of the state feel for their medical tradition; as a place of work it offers physical facilities which match the distinction of the faculty working with it.

This project of expansion had its beginning in 1939 shortly after the Doctors Mayo died. Harold Stassen, then governor of Minnesota, appointed a group of public men to the task of proposing a memorial to them. The inevitable decision was that only a further projection of their work would have gratified men who had done so much to give the benefits of modern science to the many. A medical center fully implemented with the means of care and research was surely what the Mayos would have wanted.

The Minnesota legislature, having voted unanimously to participate in the Mayo Memorial, appointed a Committee of Founders which was authorized to secure the necessary funds through public appropriations and private gifts and to arrange for a suitable memorial.

Dr. Diehl had become dean of the College of Medical Sciences in 1935 and he was eager to put into operation such plans of expansion as were envisioned by the plans for the proposed medical center. The nearly twenty-five years of Dr. Diehl's leadership covered the period when the institution achieved international reputation. His devotion to science and loyalty to both his faculty and its needs enabled him to hold together a distinguished group of men, to add frequently to their number, and to provide such conditions of work as could produce an impressive list of accomplishments. These were so widely recognized that before the end of his deanship the medical school was receiving, in addition to legislative appropriations, some two and a half million dollars annually for research. These funds came mostly from outside Minnesota. Among recent donors are the National Institutes of Health of the Public Health Service, the United States Army, the United States Navy, the Atomic Energy Commission, the Veterans' Administration, the National Research Council, the National Federation for Infantile Paralysis, the Allergy Foundation, and the American Cancer Society.

Knowing how large a constituency waited to be served, Dean Diehl wished to offer the best possible facilities for carrying out their commissions.

Fortunately, the university's staunch friend, Dr. Cowling, had accepted the chairmanship of the Committee of Founders. The history of the efforts that were required to get the Mayo Memorial actually built is a dramatic one, full of those spurts of hope, nearly calamitous reversals of fortune, and renewals of enterprise that the playwright has always loved. But the chairman was able to keep a steady hand on fate and no frustrations gave him more than a short pause for breath.

Difficulties were many. Some had to do with the changes of outlook that hamper any long-range project. These became formidable indeed when the period moved under the shadows of the Korean War and of other crises in world affairs. Appropriations from the legislature showed themselves to be woefully inadequate in the face of pressing needs and rising costs. The state's first contribution was doubled and then that sum more than tripled before the final total of $7,000,000 was reached. Even that figure was far from being high enough to build the kind of memorial the committee had planned. Federal health agencies donated $3,122,000. Individuals, corporations, and private health groups contributed an additional two and a quarter million. The roll of contributors among old and new friends of the university was long. As a final report says, it numbers "some 10,000 in Minnesota, throughout the nation and beyond."

Even with the twelve and a quarter millions in their hands, even after ground had been broken, Dr. Cowling and his committee were confronted with still greater difficulties. Another dizzy upward spiral of prices sent estimates for construction of the original model up to $15,000,000. Rather than to wait for the additional funds that another campaign might be able to supply, it was decided to complete the building with the money already raised. Careful redesigns reduced the twenty-two-story model to fourteen stories without the loss of vital features. Already some of these sacrifices have been compensated by new plans of expansion for which the legislature has supplied funds.

At the dedicatory ceremonies of the Mayo Memorial, held on the evening of October 21, 1954, Dr. Cowling reminded his audience of the place of high distinction which the Mayo brothers had gained in Minnesota history. The buildings stand, he said, "as an expression of individual and public appreciation of these preeminent citizens of our state — their zeal for truth and their eagerness to know it, their faith in unselfish ideals, their sympathy and their concern for the welfare of all men everywhere. The accomplishments of their devoted lives will continue through the ages to bless mankind."

Completion of the Mayo Memorial was not the last of Dr. Cowling's achievements in building up the medical center. As president of the Masonic Cancer Relief Committee of Minnesota and chairman of its executive committee he had a large part in helping to bring to reality the Masonic Memorial Hospital which now stands on the medical campus. Whenever the zeal of Minnesotans in the service of education is under discussion the name of Dr. Cowling will be spoken often with gratitude and pride.

The importance to the School of Nursing of the fact that it conducts its own work in intimate association with so distinguished a medical teaching and research center is obvious. The link with the College of Medical Sciences continues, of course, to be intimate. As one unit of a university system grows strong, others grow in strength, too. The school and the college have matured together and, today, the range of the ambitious plans of each stretches far wider than ever before.

In recent years the faculty of the School of Nursing has grown in numbers. As teachers have appeared who are well prepared to offer instruction, more of the work of teaching has been taken over by these members; less has been done by members of the medical faculty. However, close associations continue on every level of work. The two are vitally joined in many of their enterprises.

But the same thing may be said of the school's links to other colleges of the campus — indeed, to all the colleges. Bonds of interdependent interest exist with the College of Science, Literature and the Arts, in which nurse students earn their academic credits before entering the school; with the College of Education in which certain of its students actually take their degrees; with the School of Public Health where partnership has always been close; with the General College to which one group of students enrolled in the School of Nursing reports for courses in general education; with the Institute of Agriculture, its cosponsor of one curriculum; with the Extension Division in which its teachers conduct classes; with the Institute of Child Development and Welfare where, again, a wealth of common interests may be shared. The School of Business Administration and the Institute of Technology make valuable contributions to the program of instruction offered to nurse students. From time to time the law school cooperates by preparing mock trials, for the benefit of its own young men as well as for nurses, which illustrate problems in the legal aspects of nursing.

One of the many revealing associations of the School of Nursing with another unit of the university system is that which it maintains with the Center for Continuation Study. This "postgraduate college" was created under the leadership of President Coffman to provide a place in which men and women in the field may, from time to time, bring their techniques down to date by attending institutes which acquaint them with the latest advances in science. A full-time staff, now under the direction of Frederick E. Berger, devotes itself to the organization and presentation of short, intensive courses of instruction designed to give the practicing lawyer, doctor, nurse, teacher, social scientist a look at late developments in his field. From its beginning in November, 1936, the experiment in postgraduate education for working professionals has been highly successful. University men and women in the healing arts have used its facilities more frequently and with more continuity of effort than any other group. Dr. Harold Diehl once pointed out that the Center for Continuation Study, by offering a classroom in which the university's "strong fundamental and clinical departments" may spread the word of late discoveries, has created a medical center that has given "distinguished service not only to physicians but also to citizens of the entire region." In the same way Miss Densford and her faculty have used the center to acquaint nurses with advances in their profession. In a steady succession of institutes and workshops the School of Nursing has endorsed and furthered the philosophy that learning is not a process in which only men and women in their twenties and thirties can be expected to take an interest, but that it is, rather, one that must be encouraged to continue as long as intellectual vitality survives.

The first university School of Nursing was created at Minnesota to be part of an indivisible system of education. In the days of its early struggles for recognition there were, perhaps, those who smiled with indulgence at its desire for a place beside its august elders among the professional schools of medicine and law. Today it would be difficult to find even a vestige of that attitude. Even Woodrow Wilson failed in his 1909 discussion of the ideal university to foresee that nursing education must presently establish its claim to a permanent position in a university system. But today it has become a link in his chain, "united from end to end."

Close cooperation between the School of Nursing and the other colleges has brought from all a spontaneous understanding of the purposes of nursing education. No testimony to the importance of Katharine Densford's accomplishment could be more direct or more convincing than the respect with which the university world regards the school she has brought to maturity, the programs she has helped her faculty to develop and the broad outlook on the responsibilities of the profession which she has nurtured.

17

Citizens of the Campus

❦ A COMPOSITE portrait of the nurse student, as she looks out on the prospect of the university world today, would offer many pleasing aspects. It would show, first of all, the glow of health, the reward of the fact that, quite spontaneously she avails herself of the opportunities for swimming, skiing, figure-skating, for horseback riding, for playing tennis and golf — for every item in the long list of strenuous entertainments in which a famous vacation land abounds. It would reveal, in a certain look of expectation, that she has been alerted to the wide choice, opened to her by the lively cultural program of the campus, among the pleasures of the theater, the lecture platform, and the concert hall. It would present testimony to a sense of personal worth that belongs to a woman who knows that her world is her very own and that it is one from which she may accept any or — if she has the strength — all of a great flood of invitations to participate. The prevailing impression created by such a picture would be that of a woman contentedly poised in the midst of promises — a member of a society to which she is intimately bound by many links of mutual respect.

A second glance would show, perhaps, that this composite portrait is not very different from the portrait of a typical young woman in the arts college or the law school or on the agricultural campus. The attribute which all such pictures would have in common is a vital awareness of sharing the advantages of a good world.

It has not always been true for student nurses that they have known themselves to be valued for their contributions to the life of the community. A striking feature of the history of a school of nursing is the enormous change that it reveals in the attitude of society toward these particular members of the human family.

From the ancient days when nurses were drawn from among women of no very well defined, but generally underprivileged background, there remained in the hospital schools holdovers of a severe and humiliating discipline. Students were required to keep the hours and endure the surveillance of Victorian servants. They could expect to have no social relations with doctors. They must know their place and keep to it.

During the first decade of its existence the first university school of nursing maintained a similarly rigorous regime. As one graduate nurse has recalled, without rancor and yet without endorsement of the old ways, almost the only relaxation a student could discover lay in breaking one rule or another. It was a modest gratification to "duck out of 'Dickie' Beard's class as he was pushing a cow's heart around on a platter" and run furtively to a daytime dance in the old armory. But such pleasures were meager and they palled upon imaginations of healthy young women.

The first to protest were members of the famous class of 1919. Alma Haupt, Hortense Hilbert (Cikovsky), and Anna Jones (Mariette) constituted themselves a committee on reform. Together they went to Miss Powell and said: "We want student government." Miss Powell seemed to draw a long sigh of relief and said in effect: "Good! I have only been waiting for you to ask for it."

From that moment dates the Minnesota practice of allowing students of nursing a large measure of independence. Miss Powell herself set down for readers of the *American Journal of Nursing* the basic principles. Clearly it was wrong, she wrote, to ask students to abide by rules in the formulation of which they had had no share. Only under the protection of the democratic tradition could the human dignity of the nurse be preserved and nourished.

The foursome of Haupt, Hilbert, Jones, and McIver put their right of self-determination to immediate use. But they still limited themselves to problems of the personal life of the nurse. To give "the brown house on Church Street" a brighter look they planned many projects. The purchase of screens for an unprotected porch was made possible by giving a garden party on the lawn between the anatomy building and Millard Hall. For five cents a visitor was allowed to look at the flowers; for ten cents he might ride around the block in an automobile owned (incredibly!) by one of the girls in the nurses' home. The same group appeared before the board of regents to protest about the "unsanitary conditions" under which they were required to live. But the board briskly brushed them aside with the amused comment that their living quarters couldn't really be so bad for, surely, they were "a healthy looking crowd."

The official establishment of the Nurses' Self Government Association in 1919 was appropriately celebrated at a banquet given that year in the university hospitals. During the years when Marion Vannier was director of the School of Nursing the tradition of allowing students to take part actively in shaping their daily life developed steadily and in accordance with the generous attitudes of a wise and sympathetic woman.

But it was under the guidance of Katharine Densford that the principle of student self-government achieved the breadth of influence that it has in the affairs of the school today. Miss Densford's long record of work with the National Association of Parliamentarians, of which she was made an honorary member in 1959, and her work also as parliamentarian of the Minnesota branch of the American Association of University Women has demonstrated the sincerity of her belief in democratic procedure. But her concern went far beneath and beyond an academic knowledge of Robert's *Rules of Order*. A chief feature of her policy as administrator was to delegate authority to colleagues and then allow each delegate to evolve a program of her own design, subject only to the guidance of the will of the school as a whole. On many of the advisory committees created during her period of office, students were given representation so that they might have a voice even in matters of curriculums. The policy has been followed with so evident a desire to encourage participation that the voice of the student has grown ever stronger and is raised today with spontaneous enthusiasm in deliberations of every kind.

The N.S.G.A. has been able to stimulate a wide variety of interests within the life of the school. In 1927 it helped to bring to the campus a chapter of the national social sorority, Alpha Tau Delta, and, in 1934, a chapter of the national scholarship society, Sigma Theta Tau. Each of these has provided not merely opportunities for social intimacy among women of similar interests but also outlets for the energies of "service-centered" people in active work for welfare projects. Mixing altruism with entertainment, Alpha Tau Delta has invited guests to a succession of rummage sales, food sales, and coffee hours to raise funds for the help of such enterprises as those of the National Epilepsy League. It grants an annual scholarship, in honor of Esther M. Thompson (class of 1925), to a student in good standing registered in any of the school's programs. Sigma Theta Tau sponsors a scholarship available to any deserving student in the basic nursing course.

After more than thirty years of experience in training students for self-government the N.S.G.A. saw an opportunity, in 1951, further to expand the tradition. By dissolving its old form it was able, with the guidance of counselor Ruth V. Johnston, to transmit its spirit to new organizations which could more conveniently cover the greatly broadened area of its influence. The first of these, the Nursing College Board, is concerned with the larger affairs of the school; the second, the Powell Hall Governing Association, deals particularly with matters related to the nurses' residence.

The constitution of the N.C.B. states its purposes. They are "to foster closer and more active student-faculty relations in consideration of educational and professional matters; to promote regular studies of curricular problems, faculty-student relationships and professional and educational aims; to interchange information and to integrate the efforts of students and faculty in working toward common goals." The board is supported by dues assessed upon students of the basic professional and practical nursing programs and it recognizes the authority of the university as well as of the Senate Committee on Student Affairs.

Earnest as its intentions are, the board does not suffocate these in an atmosphere of blue-stocking intensity. Its interests include such a steady round of "mixers," coffee hours, and fireside hours as would make Miss Powell both glad and envious. It entertains speakers who are invited to discuss either aspects of the nurse's professional work or subjects of general interest to a woman of the modern world. It acts as recruitment agency for the school by including in many of its entertainments students from the arts college who may find the atmosphere sympathetic and decide to enroll. It has sent a student to the International Council of Nurses holding its quadrennial congress in a far-distant place. It has, in recent years, adopted a German war orphan and, in a long-term program of benevolence, assured the child's education.

The extracurricular program of the school, as a thoughtful and varied display of the opportunities offered by human experience, can have left few avenues unexplored. Within the walls of Powell Hall the social life of the community is as different as possible from the meager outlook faced by Miss Powell when she had almost to beg for $12 with which to give an occasional party in Shevlin. Myrtle Gagnon, director for a long time, had the privilege — and used it well — of lending an expert's talents to the design of recreation for the nursing student. Now that Miss Gagnon has moved to a new scene of undergraduate social life on the St. Paul campus, she has been succeeded by Esther B. Hayes, who will practice what Miss Powell preached so long: that the exercise of the play spirit is not only a legitimate activity in student life but one that is absolutely essential to the full development of creative intelligence.

But the outlook of nurse students is by no means limited to what may be seen from the windows of Powell Hall. Energetic as life within the nurses' residence would seem to be, it does not exhaust the vitality of the occupants. Their vigor surges far beyond to leap over old barriers and touch every phase of student activity. Members of the school are, in every sense, citizens of the campus. An official link is established by representation on the All-University Congress. But this is only the foundation of an active concern with campus politics, campus social life, campus philanthropy, and, in general, campus ferment. Student nurses have served in such elective jobs as that of membership on the Board of Governors for Coffman Memorial Union. They apply for, and get, appointments to organizations like the Board in Control of Student Publications (or Board of Pub, as the undergraduate, displaying his happy gifts for abbreviation and impudence, has learned to call it). They work on-stage or backstage in the numerous productions of the university theater. They sing in the university chorus. Much more actively than many another less close-knit group they participate in such spectacles as the Carnival, an annual event which lends the brilliantly garish color of the circus to campus life, exploiting fully student wit and student ingenuity. Student nurses have been candidates for campus queen whenever the impulse to create royalty seizes on the democratic imagination of the undergraduate.

Because they are, as a group, seriously concerned with the problem of increasing enrollment in their profession, student nurses are always to be found in the midst of those projects which undertake to recommend the university to incoming students. At freshman camp and during orientation week they proselytize cheerfully and eloquently. At the State Fair they sometimes maintain a booth in which are displayed evidences of the advances recently made by their profession and, just incidentally, attractions to possible students. Whenever citizens of the campus are enlisted to help in raising money for local or national projects such as the Community Chest or drives for the support of research in cancer, cerebral palsy, or multiple sclerosis, student nurses are numerically strong among them. Because of their special orientation they are likely to be vigorous also in eloquence. Further evidence that these students are no less representative in their seriousness than in their ebullience may be found in the fact that many are enrolled in one or another of the numerous religious organizations on the campus.

Like Ariel, the student nurse is everywhere. Whether it is in a Greek-letter sorority, in a group organized for folk dancing, or in the Rooter's Club, identification with the round of university occupations, pastimes, and pleasures is complete and satisfying.

It is chiefly the student in the basic professional course who finds within herself the excess energy to give to this exhausting parade of activities. Candidates for advanced degrees find themselves preoccupied, as do students in other colleges of the campus, with the exacting requirements of their academic work. Some are employed as dormitory nurses or in other part-time jobs. However, the scores of scholarships, fellowships, traineeships, and stipends now available to candidates of high standing offer a large measure of support. These come from a variety of sources: the faculty of the school itself, the National League for Nursing, the Minnesota Department of Public Welfare, but most particularly from the national government through the army, the navy, or the United States Public Health Service. Awareness at Washington of a need to encourage the training of the nurse at a high level for the protection and care of its citizens has made the daily life of the student nurse strikingly different from any condition that Florence Nightingale, or even Isabel Hampton Robb, would be able to recognize. As a result of the 1956 Health Amendments Act, passed by the Congress, traineeships for the year 1956–57 amounting to $107,744 and in 1957–58 amounting to $134,212 were assigned to the University of Minnesota School of Nursing for the preparation of nurse educators and administrators.

The student nurse is no less conscious than are men and women enrolled in other colleges on the campus that she lives in a center of quite

unusual cultural activity. The Cyrus Northrop Memorial Auditorium
is the home of the Minneapolis Symphony Orchestra which, during the
past quarter of a century, has been conducted in succession by Eugene
Ormandy, Dimitri Mitropoulos, and Antal Dorati. It has provided the
setting in several seasons past for presentations of the Metropolitan
Opera Company, and is regularly used for the recitals of the University
Artists Course. The student nurse may attend such events at the reduced
prices available to all citizens of the campus. But even if the price still
does not fit her pocketbook, she simply exchanges her white uniform for
a black and white one and hears Tebaldi, Rubinstein, or Menuhin as
an usher, perched on the stairs.

"The great voices of the time" are audible to her. Lectures highlight
the calendar of each week of the year, twelve months long. With other
undergraduates and graduates she attends these occasions with a sober
concern for opportunity which testifies incontestably to the maturity of
the present-day population of the campus. Northrop Auditorium a few
years ago proved to be inadequate — though its seating capacity is nearly
5,000 — to house the audience assembled to hear T. S. Eliot speak on the
frontiers of literary criticism, and the devotees of poetry had to be
moved to Williams arena, which is more usually host to basketball fans.
On less startling occasions of recent years the hall has proved to be just
large enough to receive those gathered to hear such representatives of
public life, the arts, the sciences, and the social sciences as William O.
Douglas, Ralph Bunche, the late Thomas Mann, John Gielgud, Van-
nevar Bush, and Arnold Toynbee.

Possibly as a result, in part, of the fact that she has had these stimulating exposures to the best intelligences of the world, the Minnesota
nurse has become increasingly aware of international responsibilities.
In 1955, at the suggestion of Katharine Densford, Phyllis Halvorson, a
senior student at Minnesota and president of the National Student
Nurses' Association, put before that body a proposal for the creation of
an international student nurses' organization. Its purposes: to foster
international good will; to provide a medium for the exchange of ideas;
to encourage among students an interest in developments within their
profession throughout other countries; and to promote the interests of
student nurses everywhere. The American Nurses Association acted
favorably when the student association presented the idea and recommended its adoption by the International Council of Nurses. This or-

ganization, in turn, acted favorably and the International Student Nurses' Unit was authorized in 1957.

The modern nurse lives in an atmosphere which tends to make it impossible for her to be provincial. The International Council of Nurses, created in 1899, is the oldest organization of professional women. Student nurses who are now invited to develop their individual philosophies in the reflected light of so august a parent group can hardly fail to become women of the world in the best modern sense.

Alumnae of the school are active in all the ways that are appropriate to their responsibility as graduates of an excellent school and to their pride as representatives of a school with great prestige. They are active, first of all, in posts of importance all around the world. Lucile Petry Leone has offered the standing bet that if she were to be dropped by parachute on an unknown town anywhere in the country she would appear, within twenty-four hours, leading a nurse who had been trained at Minnesota. It would take her longer, perhaps, to find one on a distant outpost of civilization anywhere on the globe. But given time and a plane she would probably return with her mission accomplished, for Minnesota women have gone on overseas assignments to Korea, Iraq, Tripoli, India, Iran, and almost every place in the world that a geographer, trying conscientiously to be baffling, could name.

The Minnesota Nurses' Alumnae Association maintains a close link with the activities of the school today. In the past it has been independent of other organizations of university graduates; it has published its own magazine and been sole sponsor of its own events such as the annual banquet. One of its activities is to raise funds for the endowment of the school initiated by Dr. Beard. Now that the potential membership has grown very large — nearly four thousand — the group has voted to work chiefly through two agencies that will help to give its plans a broader reach. Members of the Alumnae Association have become constituent members of the General Alumni Association of the university and that able organization will support its purposes. Benefactions of the alumnae will be administered through the newly established University of Minnesota School of Nursing Foundation.

However, the association continues to exercise a direct influence on the interests of the school. A recent contribution to the preservation of tradition in a warmly personal way was that of commissioning Edward

Brewer to paint a portrait of Katharine Densford which now hangs in Powell Hall. At the unveiling a spokesman of the association commented on the appropriateness of this tribute. Her image will serve to remind former students of how much she has done to "keep us proud to be alumnae of the school." Further to mark its "gratitude and high esteem" the association awarded to Miss Densford, upon her retirement, its "Certificate of Merit."

That moment of familial pride was well earned. For Katharine Densford, her faculty, and her graduates have, through their influence, almost literally "put a girdle round the earth."

18

Tomorrow Is a Comer

IN ONE of his many brisk challenges to the creative spirit of American democracy, Carl Sandburg warns that there should be no looking backward because, as he says, "Yesterday is a goner." To a vigorous interpreter of Sandburg's kind the statement carries the implication that tomorrow is a "comer." It is quite possible to conceive of tomorrow as a leaden-footed giant approaching with a great bungling bundle of apprehensions. It is equally possible to regard it as a "crusader of light" flashing hope into the dark corners of human society. The American professions seem determined to take the hopeful view. Certainly the profession of nursing reflects in all its literature a readiness to seize the opportunities, lately opened up by science, and put them to work to improve the human condition.

Nursing, as a profession and an art, asks and expects many things of the future.

First of all, it wants numbers, because now, more than ever before, in numbers there is strength. The supply of nurses has never been adequate and in our generation, when much more is expected of the nurse than in any previous one, the force is far below what it should be. The National League for Nursing estimates that there are 480,000 of their company in the United States today. By 1970 there should be from 600,000 to 700,000. The profession wants a higher ratio of nurses to population. For every 100,000 citizens there are now 258 nurses. To improve service, as both the public and the profession wish urgently to see it improved, that ratio should rise at least to 300 per 100,000. In more nearly ideal circumstances it would rise to 350 per 100,000. The means must be found by which many more students can be recruited. And they must be held within the profession not because of their individual altruism but because their education and vocation are such that their self-respect will be nourished. The professional status of the nurse has been established thanks, in part, to the pioneering effort at the University of Minnesota. A more general acknowledgment of her status as a professional worker on a high level, with a multiplicity of fascinating but exacting duties to perform, each requiring specialized instruction – this should help to bring into the profession the large company of alert, earnest, adaptable intelligences that it needs.

Second, the nursing profession wants for all its members more complete, more flexible, more effectively administered programs and procedures of instruction. It is no longer reasonable to expect representatives of hospital staffs and hard-driven men of medical faculties, whose chief concern is with other areas of teaching, to provide classroom and laboratory instruction in all the wide variety of subjects which make up the modern curriculum of nursing. The unquestionably great advantage of close cooperation between medical school and school of nursing can no longer be made to cover all needs in a complex organization like that of a great university. The days of homespun improvisation are gone – gone, one might say, with the winds that roar through the atomic age. A present-day school of nursing needs an adequate basic faculty of its own.

Third, the nursing profession needs women with advanced preparation. Even today there are far too few graduate nurses with training beyond the bachelor's level. Consequently the supply of nurses fitted to fill teaching jobs and administrative positions is far below demand. Announcements of vacancies in such fields fall, not upon deaf ears, but upon the ears of women who know themselves to be insufficiently prepared for such responsibilities. And the posts remain unfilled to the great detriment of hospital efficiency. Since the economy of the country still produces few women who can afford to support themselves of their own efforts, or with family assistance, beyond the four or five years required of all candidates for the bachelor of science degree, fellowships for advanced study must be made available to particularly able people, and these must be large enough to enable the graduate nurse to devote herself exclusively to academic work, free of the strain of having to earn tuition and living expense at an outside job. The United States government has recognized the importance of the problem by creating trainee-ships for the preparation of teachers and administrators, but the need remains to provide for such benefits on a continuing basis. In today's battle for survival, opponents of our own ideals have tended to trans-form education into a weapon of offense. No country can afford, in such a crisis, to regard education merely as a decorative shield.

Fourth, the nursing profession wants to encourage research in its own field. No sign of maturity in an educational institution is so unmistak-able or so reassuring as the desire to share in the responsibilities of this field. Many such research activities already exist. Joint and cooperative projects in which nurses participate have to do with such important problems as mental health, the treatment of cancer, neurological condi-tions, infectious diseases, allergies, arthritis, and metabolic disorders. More studies of the kind are needed. The School of Nursing at Minne-sota wants a faculty that is qualified — and has time — to serve as effec-tive members of research teams in the field of health and human welfare.

The many large-scale, often history-making, medical researches that have been conducted at the University of Minnesota during the past twenty years have inspired the enthusiasm of nurses who assist in them. On their own initiative teachers and students alike have begun to ask for advance information about new operations and new treatments, so that they may prepare for the best possible performance of their own roles. They ask not merely for recognition as members of the team, but that they be given new responsibilities.

In the past it has been the practice of the great foundations, in plan-ning large projects which universities are asked to carry out, to account in their budgets for every foreseeable need — except nursing. But now at long last a breakthrough toward establishing a new tradition seems to have come. A new long-range research project at Minnesota has at the start an appropriation for nursing service.

This is part of the nationwide collaborative study established in 1957 by the National Institute of Neurological Diseases and Blindness with the support of Congress. The purpose is to investigate the relation-ship between factors and conditions affecting parents and the occur-rence in their offspring of such conditions as cerebral palsy and mental retardation. The medical center at the University of Minnesota is one of fourteen participating in the project. The scope of its investigations is broad, and at Minnesota the project is now known as the Child Development Study. Nurses are playing an increasingly important role in it. Since January, 1958, Mrs. Harriet Morgart, who earned her baccalaureate degree and a master in nursing education degree at Minnesota and who was formerly a member of the faculty of the school, has been an instructor in the department of pediatrics. Her team, which now consists of six research nurses, will assist in gathering data.

This sort of admission to full partnership in the work of investigation is another trend which the nursing profession would like to encourage in the hope of seeing the health work of the world performed with the deftness that the brilliance of recent medical discoveries should inspire.

A fifth proposal which leaders of the nursing profession sponsor today is that the work of conserving human life and human resources should be conducted on an international basis. Well-being must become possible for all people everywhere if it is to be the secure possession of any people anywhere.

The Minnesota community has assumed the responsibility of putting this idea to work. In 1954, at the special urging of a Minnesota alumnus, Harold Stassen, the university accepted an assignment from the Foreign Operations Administration of the United States government to help rehabilitate the educational facilities of Seoul National University, devastated by the Korean War. Representatives of Minnesota's Institute of Agriculture, its Institute of Technology, and its College of Medical Sciences went out to replace guns with equipment for laboratories and classrooms. It was their task to advise and help in the advancement of curriculums and teaching methods so that a people who had been plagued for forty years by the oppressive weight of dictatorship could take up and carry forward the job of operating their own way of life in peace and dignity. At the same time Korean educators came to Minnesota to refresh their understanding of public health precepts, clouded so long by war's appalling shadow. Among them were Mrs. Kwi Hyang Lee, director of the school of nursing at Seoul University and Miss Song Hi Lee, its surgical nursing instructor. Miss Yeo Shin Hong, instructor of introductory nursing, arrived in Minnesota in 1958. Overcoming the language barrier by learning English in speeded-up classes, these women acquired a knowledge of new techniques by which the Koreans could utilize the discoveries of modern science.

The university also sent its representatives to Korea. Among them was Margery Low of the School of Nursing faculty. Carrying with her the school's philosophy that care of the patient is the primary concern of all health projects, she worked with the hospital nurses for the improvement of nursing; she worked also with the faculty to upgrade the program of the school itself. New equipment has been purchased for the hospital at Seoul which had been stripped by the Communists of every valuable and useful object. A "Help Korea" train carried some $16,000 worth of supplies for the school alone: beds, mattresses, scales, obstetric manikins, syringes, intravenous apparatus, a catalogue which reads — if its overtone of sympathetic understanding be heard — less like a listing of equipment than like a paean in praise of the spirit of international responsibility.

Miss Low was succeeded in 1958 by Joan Williams.

A similiar demonstration of the fraternal temper which exists throughout the modern world of science took place in the city of Minneapolis in 1958. The Tenth Anniversary Special Commemorative Session of the World Health Assembly and the eleventh WHO Assembly meetings were held there during the last days of May and the first of June. To it eighty-eight nations sent representatives. They came from every corner of the globe speaking a diversity of tongues, wearing a diversity of costumes, and embodying the traditions of a diversity of cultures. But the significance of the occasion, like that of all the other conferences brought together by WHO, lay in the fact that there was complete agreement on the purpose of the gathering which, as its literature said, was to promote the concept of health as "a complete state of physical, mental and social well-being — not merely the absence of disease."

Among the participants there were many nurses. Katharine Densford served as chief representative of the International Council of Nurses. Many members of the profession were present from Austria, Colombia, Israel, Japan, Liberia, the Netherlands, the Philippines, and the United Kingdom to carry back to their national organizations word of the proceedings. Many more came as individual observers to attend sessions in the public galleries. All were prompted by the conviction, held as tenet number one in the philosophy of the nursing profession today, that only through international cooperation can the purposes of health care be accomplished.

As a springboard to the future the School of Nursing has recently set in motion the propulsive power of a new organization. The University of Minnesota School of Nursing Foundation, which came into being on November 15, 1958, will undertake to bring to reality the school's ambitious plans. These have specifically to do with the further development of undergraduate and graduate programs; the expansion of provisions for financial aid to students; the improvement of such aids to education as audiovisual techniques; the enrichment of opportunity for students by the creation of lectureships and through a broadened faculty exchange program; providing means by which faculty and staff may attend professional meetings, workshops, and conferences; offering assistance in the publication of research findings and useful papers read at conferences; helping to support the desire of faculty members to take leaves of absence for further study; encouraging research of every kind.

A group of public-spirited citizens are endorsers of the plan. Prominent among them is Mrs. Walter W. Walker, who is serving as president for the first three years. Another is Mrs. Frank Bowman, who has always been a faithful friend of the school, one upon whom it could count, as it would count on Mrs. Walker, for support of every kind.

Direction of the affairs of the foundation will be in the hands of a board of directors representing the alumnae of the school, educators, and the general public. Ex-officio members will be the president of the university, the dean of the College of Medical Sciences, the director of the school, the director of the hospitals, the director of nursing services, and the director of the Greater University Fund.

In the past it has been an important part of the responsibility of the school's director to find funds for necessary activities which the budget could not support. These have come from the great foundations, from the United States government, and from private benefactors. The director who voluntarily assumed this task pursued its aims for nearly thirty years with a resourcefulness, a knowledge of her field, and a tactful persuasiveness which has set an example for missionary workers of the kind.

But the stress of many urgent needs has made it clear that, in the future, such time-consuming and uncertain methods of fund-raising must be replaced by a modern instrument of benefaction. Like other agencies of its kind, the School of Nursing Foundation will undertake to stimulate giving from many sources; it will utilize the donations it receives to further the purposes of health care with the utmost economy of means, avoiding duplication of effort and making room for the adaptation to the requirements of future generations of the fundamental intent of nursing education. The establishment of the foundation, accomplished by Katharine Densford and the members of her faculty, summarizes the effort of thirty years. It will help to organize their ambitions for the school and to make their realization practicable.

Two of the purposes of the foundation — "to offer assistance in the publication of useful papers" and "to promote research of every kind" — will help to satisfy needs of which the nursing profession has been conscious for almost three quarters of a century. The message from Florence Nightingale, read before the conference of nurses at the World's Columbian Exposition at Chicago in 1893, called attention to the lack of nursing literature. Forty years later, Dr. May Ayres Burgess was still disturbed about its meagerness. The body of printed work was pitifully undernourished, she said; there was "little about techniques, next to nothing about hospital administration . . . research, unknown." Her tone was almost that of one crying in the wilderness.

Today that wilderness has been explored, intensively developed, and put in civilized order. Its field of study has been systematically cultivated and made to yield important products for the use of the profession. The world of nurses sounds with the voices of vigorous-minded women who know what they know and are eager to communicate their knowledge. Grateful for the acknowledgment of their professional status, rejoicing in the fact that they have been accepted as partners in the work of healing, as well as in the tasks of patient care, they have seized upon the highest responsibility of scholarship, which is to make original contribution to the investigation of problems.

This literature now grows rapidly and to its wealth alumnae of the first university school of nursing have made many contributions. The steady, helpful pressure made by Katharine Densford on the members of her faculty to work for advanced degrees has resulted in the production of many doctoral dissertations which have strengthened the body of knowledge. Among those who have made such investigations are Helen Nahm, now dean of the school of nursing at the University of California; Rena Boyle, now head of the Nursing and Consultation branch of the Division of Nursing Resources, Public Health Service, Washington, D.C.; Myrtle Kitchell Aydelotte, professor and former dean of the College of Nursing at the State University of Iowa; Isabel

Harris, now assistant to the director of Minnesota's own school; and the late Ruth V. Johnston.

Expert as teachers, these women have used their gifts of communication to add to the resources of nursing information and understanding. They have satisfied the definition of research offered by the *American Journal of Nursing* in December, 1950: "The orderly, systematic collection of facts and the classification, analysis and interpretation of those facts in relation to a specific problem."

And in doing so they have helped to escort their profession into the world of tomorrow.

Postscript and Prelude

🌿 A span of fifty years measures different prospects for different observers. To the young time seems to stretch on and on with the awe-inspiring promise and the awful threat of eternity. To the old the period encompasses the effort of a lifetime with all its hopes and disappointments, its frustrations and fulfillments. In the eye of a historian like Professor Toynbee, who takes the formidable record of human destiny and all the falls and rises of civilization as his field, half a century is likely to represent at most a searching glance and more usually a mere somnolent blink.

Yet the particular period measured in the academic way from July of 1909 to June of 1959 covers a time of significant change in the outlook for humanity. That the outlook is both better and worse than it was fifty years ago no reader of the daily newspaper could fail to agree. Such a follower of human affairs may comfort himself with the thought that, however much certain prospects have darkened in the dust of conflict, others have brightened in the light of science.

Education, alerted by the noble insights of the past when all the eternal verities were declared, has moved forward at an eager pace during the past half century, using new techniques for the coordination of knowledge and new tools for the exact measurement of probabilities. In particular, education for health has improved far beyond the imagining of a world that continued to be ancient in method until the enormous effort of research began.

Narrowing the field of vision a little further, it is evident that education for nursing has completely changed its character in fifty years. In the early years of the century the work of the nurse was still regarded as little better than a menial task. The workers themselves were likely to consider it as a mere occupation, a livelihood that was useful to a young woman as she moved away from the dependence of childhood and toward the security of marriage.

In half a century nursing has moved out of the deep shadow of its immemorial past and emerged as a profession. Able women who saw both its possibilities and its responsibilities insisted rigorously on a re-examination of attitudes, on a reappraisal of purposes, on improvement of method in instruction, on a refounding of the whole educational system. Under the unremittent prodding of leaders, working through the national organizations which they had helped to create, the profession came of age. Its techniques were revised and strengthened; its standards made firm and solid. Reaching maturity with the encouragement of the same vigorous preceptresses, the profession used its national publications to urge the establishment of better schools, ones in which the content of curriculums would be deepened by study of the sciences, broadened by the knowledge and use of each improvement in method as it came along. Knowing that no school can be better than its teachers, the profession insisted on the introduction into curriculums of courses particularly designed to train those who must train others. In the bulletins of leading institutions, offerings for advanced clinical study appeared and, soon after, programs for graduate study. In fifty years nursing had rehearsed the whole story of the march of education toward high ground. And not the least significant aspect of its steadily sustained program was the demand that by careful methods of recruitment and selection schools of nursing should discover and mine resources of superior human material. The records of students' achievement prove that, in this, as in the other phases of its campaign for self-improvement, the profession has been conspicuously successful.

To this history the School of Nursing at Minnesota has made many important contributions in each division of effort and on all levels of accomplishment. The position of influence held by its director in the councils of nurses insured to the school a vital place of leadership. She knew where able people were to be found. She attracted such women to her faculty; she made a principle of opening the windows of all the minds with which she was associated on the broadest possible view of the nurse's work; she gave voice to the young and had faith in the proposals of new faculty members even when these were untried — perhaps *particularly* when these were untried. With her faculty she developed programs of instruction which have become models for directors of other institutions to follow. Often in the course of an administration covering nearly thirty years she had the experience of sending a teacher who had profited conspicuously by this generous treatment to a position of large creative responsibility in a realm needing such service. She sent them regretfully yet with that blend of graciousness, earnestness, and pride that has always characterized her outlook. The faculty, she has always insisted, "made the school." As servants of a difficult but hopeful discipline they must go where there were still worlds to make or to remake in the image of healthy promise. Of the thousands who were graduated from the school in Miss Densford's time, hundreds have gone to key positions as directors of important schools, as officials of government services, as consultants to health agencies in every corner of the world.

To students, faculty, and fellow consultants in national and international councils, Miss Densford has always undertaken to impart a positive, creative philosophy for the profession. To her, nursing means not merely the healing of a wound but it includes the idea of taking foresight so that wounds may not be inflicted. It means not alone the care of disease but the conquering of disease itself. It means not simply wishing a patient godspeed at the hospital door but following him home to set in motion those influences of complete rehabilitation which theoretical science has been at such pains to explore and to understand. It means to recognize realistically, if grimly, that the world today presents hitherto unimagined dangers from war, disaster, tensions, and pressures, the effects of which must be anticipated and, as far as possible, averted. It means that as all the circumstances of daily living become, moment by moment, more complex, nursing must be prepared to turn the lights of insight, of resourcefulness, of instruction into all the dark corners of these complexities. It must be ready to cope with dangers in all their physical and psychological manifestations. It must lend its invaluable and irreplaceable assistance to the end not merely of preserving life but of preserving the promises of life which are, ironically, brighter and better than ever before even at this moment when civilization itself is gravely threatened.

It was inevitable that the celebration of the school's fiftieth anniversary, held in June, 1959, should have been made an occasion not for looking back complacently at the past but for an eager examination of the outlook for the future. The Forward Look was the over-all name given to the week's session of lectures, discussions, roundtables, concerts, theatrical performances, and banquets.

It is significant that the creators of the program found it appropriate to hold not one conference but two. The first was concerned with the consideration of new practices in nursing; the other with the study of how nursing may profit by use of "the arts and skills of a liberal education." No narrow specialist, the nurse of today wishes to emphasize for herself and for newcomers to the profession the belief that, though professional knowledge makes up the bulk of her equipment, this would be meager if it left out awareness of other values and other agents of healing. The conference, called Perception and Professional Nursing, suggested the many ways in which the play spirit and the undying impulse to create may be evoked to persuade the body and mind to renounce the habit of illness and to welcome health.

The clinical conference was concerned with topics the importance of which must have been almost as evident to readers of the science columns in the daily newspaper as they were to specialists. Experts in various fields — and in some instances creators of new techniques — described such matters of universal interest as open-heart surgery, the use of the artificial kidney, new forms of psychiatric therapy, the fight against cancer, the value of antibiotics in the prevention and treatment of rheumatic fever, new drugs in the treatment of hypertension. The look, from the vantage point of a medical center where experiments and researches of many kinds are actually in progress, was far forward, indeed.

Even the concert with which the celebration began offered no merely formal salute to culture. Its effectiveness lay, in part, in the fact that nursing was its theme and nurses were among its active participants. Paul Oberg, of the university's department of music, directed an orchestra, the members of which were all borrowed from the Minneapolis Symphony Orchestra. The second half of the program consisted of the contributions of a huge choir made up of twelve choruses severally organized in nursing schools of Minnesota. One of their numbers, a Hymn and Benediction, was especially composed for the occasion by William Collins who took his inspiration from two poems written to celebrate the nurse's role in healing. The readiness and the ability to dramatize the occasion in terms of art would have been impressive in themselves: the beauty of the hymn and the distinguished style with which it was presented made the whole performance moving and memorable.

The play was another accomplishment of similar kind. It, too, was especially written for the occasion by Lowell Manfull, a member of the faculty of the university theater. "The Light in the Deepening Dark" retold the story of Edith Cavell, an English nurse who during World War I cared for the wounded of all nationalities in a Belgian hospital. She was executed by the German forces on the charge, to which she freely admitted, of having helped English soldiers to escape capture. Nurse Cavell's only defense was that of saying, in effect, that her cause was the cause of life, not of death. The authentic scene of her serene calm as she awaited martyrdom introduced into the play a final passage of great power. Scrupulously drained of easy eloquence and of theatricality in the ordinary sense, the theme was handled by the playwright with so sure a hold on genuine sentiment and so reserved, yet searching, a sense of drama that it fulfilled the purpose of tragedy which is to uplift the mind by contemplation of the finest values of the human spirit. No more appropriate tribute to the tradition of nursing at its most dedicated and sacrificial could have been found.

At the banquet, given in Coffman Memorial Union, nearly seven hundred alumnae and friends of the school were tactfully led out of any possible impulse to turn the rites into those of obsequy by the fortunate gaiety of Lucile Petry Leone's tone in the role of mistress of ceremonies. Because the occasion coincided with Katharine Densford's final appearance at a large social gathering as director of the school there were many salutes to her thirty-year record of significant contributions to the improvement of nursing education. All were spoken by the president of the university and the others in terms of warm, personal admiration for a woman who, as she "retires," will actually broaden once more her outlook on the responsibility of the nurse toward her profession.

Again the session was one arranged by nurses, conducted by nurses for the ever-growing company of the friends of nursing. It ended with a pageant dramatizing the school's history, the commentary of which was beautifully spoken by Dorothy Titt of the school's faculty. The concluding feature was a symbolic dance composition performed by three young students of the school.

There were other occasions to mark the nurses' week. At a convocation on May 7, Dr. Charles Mayo, son of the university's benefactor and himself a regent, spoke on the forward look of all the healing arts. Five graduates of the school were presented with the university's Distinguished Achievement Award: Colonel Frances I. Lay, chief of the Air Force Nurse Corps; Colonel Inez Haynes, chief of the Army Nurse Corps; Myrtle Kitchell Aydelotte, professor and former dean of the college of nursing at the State University of Iowa; Rena Boyle, chief of the branch of consultation and research, United States Public Health Service; and Mildred Montag, professor in the division of nursing education at Teachers College, Columbia University.

On Minnesota's Cap and Gown day it is the traditional practice to announce honors for all students of the university. These are recorded in the program and acknowledged from the platform as the recipients stand. There are nowadays too many to make individual recognition possible. But it is still the students' special day even though the distinguished ones among them must be saluted in a body.

It is also traditional to ask a member of the faculty who has served long and honorably and who is about to retire to make the address. At the Cap and Gown day celebration held on May 21, 1959, the choice was Katharine Densford. It was the first time in the history of the university that a woman had been so honored.

Miss Densford's subject was "You and the World of Tomorrow." Again she emphasized, as for three decades she had done in consultations with one student, with a group of three, or of three thousand, the belief that the assets brought together by university training must be turned back to society in the form of service.

An earlier gathering had anticipated all these others. Mention of it is reserved for the end of this postscript because it was the only one at which the impulse toward eulogy was permitted to indulge itself unchecked by the reticent director. This was a dinner honoring Miss Densford, given on April 23, 1959, in the Coffman Memorial Union under the auspices of the nursing organizations and the faculty. At it, the dean of the College of Medical Sciences, members of the faculty of the school, associates in nursing organizations and in public life, students of the school — all offered testimony. It was made clear that, in the collective mind of coworkers and friends, the image of Katharine Densford will be more surely enduring even than the portrait of her that hangs in

Powell Hall. Witnesses from far places who could not attend the dinner also sent their gifts of the spirit — no others were permitted — in writing.

To one of these observers Katharine Densford personified the spirit of the ideal American nurse — "intelligent, handsome, regal and friendly — all this her ordinary, everyday self." Another remembered her gratefully for the fact that she had always "brought out the best in her faculty . . . And that best has gone around the world." A third was impressed by the fact that her interest "in promoting health had resulted in better understanding between American and foreign nurses."

Mildred Montag expressed fully Miss Densford's right to a permanent place on the roster of academic leadership in her profession.

As head of one of the best known university programs in nursing, you have been in the forefront of new ideas whether it was in pioneering in the preparation of practical nurses or in developing better teachers, supervisors and administrators. Always you kept the care of the patient as focal point for students and faculty. One of your outstanding contributions has been emphasized in the full development of the potential of the individual. The world is richer for the young men and women who have been inspired by your guidance.

And it remained for Daisy C. Bridges, general secretary of the International Council of Nurses, to express the personal view: "There can be few nurses who are so widely known and loved for ready help, wise guidance and gaiety of spirit."

These are fitting tributes to an influence that has been as pervasive as it has been practical, as urgent as it has been gentle, as immediate as the day's need and as full of vision as dedication to the ideal of enduring service could make it. Happily these votes of confidence were addressed to a woman who is handsome and vigorous, one who walks toward the future with a brisk step as though toward a new assignment of the utmost interest, challenge, and excitement. Those who know Miss Densford well have no doubt that she will carry always the enormous tote bag that has become her mark of identification; that in it she will file the records of much pressing business in hand; and that, as she travels in the interest, perhaps, of international understanding among nurses, all this business will be conducted with authority and dispatch. In whatever tasks she may give herself, Miss Densford's intimates agree, thousands will benefit by her work and thousands more will enjoy personal association with her.

One of her faculty members has recalled that whenever, in the past, an attempt was made to speak to Miss Densford of a problem solved or a hope fulfilled, she would dismiss any compliment with the comment: "But, my dear, there are still so many things to do." Katharine Densford will have to wait long for an epitaph but, in the end, it may well be this: The reminder to the world that there are still so many things to do.

Dramatizing, with characteristically modest emphasis, the lifelong belief that the end of one career should mark the inauguration of another, Miss Densford, only a month after her retirement from the faculty of the university, married. On August 8, 1959, she became the wife of Carl Arminius Dreves of St. Paul.

Educated as a lawyer, Mr. Dreves had been, for many years, head of a food brokerage firm. At the same time he had been active in humanitarian movements of civic, national, and international scope. Following his retirement from business, he had devoted his time with great energy to these interests — such, for example, as attending sessions of the International Church Conference in Germany, as delegate of the Evangelical and Reformed Church.

Sharing a preoccupation with the social interests of the world community, Mr. and Mrs. Dreves, since their marriage, have joined their energies in support of a common concern for the advancement of international understanding in the fields of science, religion, and education. Mrs. Dreves, though she has resigned from all major administrative responsibilities, continues to travel widely, with her husband — writing, speaking, and consulting in many realms of nursing activity. She is, at present, serving as the nurse national co-chairman of a fund campaign sponsored by the American Nurses' Foundation, aimed at raising within the current year a sum of one million dollars to support projects for research in nursing.

In the life of a vigorous institution there can never be any break longer than the familiar one "for station identification." The station which the School of Nursing has reached is a fortunate one but, as any reader of the record must understand, that cannot justify loitering in its pleasant shade. A postscript to the history of fifty years must be simply a prelude to the next fifty and the fifty after that.

Already the future is in sight. Recently adopted regulations will make the conduct of affairs simpler though this simplicity, to be sure, imposes new duties. It has to do with the selection of students.

From its earliest days the school has exercised the right to receive only promising students. Standards have always been kept high. In a farewell note to her present activities the director of the school thanked the state of Minnesota for sending her "a most able group of students," pointing out that in the graduating class for the year 1958–59, ten of the forty-six members had stood either first or second in their high school classes and more than half had been in the upper ten per cent. To safeguard standards more securely still the school will, in the future, admit only a selected group of "affiliating" students. As of January 1, 1959, the regulation reads, they will be accepted only from college or university programs, no longer from the diploma programs of the three-year schools.

Routine will be better disciplined by the decision, recently accepted by university authorities, that beginning in 1959–60 only one class will be enrolled each year. Instead of entering at different breaks in the academic calendar, students must enter in the fall quarter. Scheduling of classes, arrangement for field service — everything that has to do with the planning of programs — will benefit from this one item of progress for which the school has worked long.

Most important of all, the ancient problem of the "apprentice system" has been resolved. At Minnesota an end will soon come to the practice of offering the student nurse instruction in return for service (with board and lodging added). Candidates for degrees in nursing will enter the university as do students in any other college. They will pay tuition and receive education in return. They will not be assigned for experience in the hospitals for 56 hours a week as they were in the distant past, nor for 42 hours as they were in a later period nor even for a maximum of 30 hours as they are today. Instead they will report there only as their schedules of instruction require them to do. This revolution has long been urged by the National League for Nursing. Certain universities already have put it into effect. Thanks to the generous policy and understanding of the university, the principle has been adopted for the Minnesota school and will become operative in the year 1961–62.

As the prospect for the coming years unfolds new faces appear among those who will guide the affairs of the school. In 1958 the University of

Minnesota made its reluctant farewell to Dr. Harold Diehl, long dean of the College of Medical Sciences. Because of his unique experience and background in the work for public health, very particularly for his brilliant achievements in furthering the fight against cancer, he was drafted to become senior vice-president of the American Cancer Society, charged with the important responsibility, already so familiar to him, of coordinating efforts in research. To his place has come Dr. Robert B. Howard, a young man who has crowded into less than four decades the activities of a normal lifetime. He earned his M.D. (1945) and Ph.D. (1952) at the University of Minnesota. He has been a captain in the medical corps, a teacher of medicine in his alma mater, its director of postgraduate medical education, and before his new appointment, associate dean. His predecessor has spoken of the high regard in which Dr. Howard is held by physicians of the state and of the Northwest for "his imaginative and enthusiastic leadership and his friendly effective cooperation." In introducing him to the large community he will now serve, Dr. Diehl has added a note of personal appreciation for "his keen and active mind, his earnestness, idealism and resourcefulness, his dedication to the job and his warm, friendly personality."

Miss Ruth Harrington served ably as acting director pending the arrival of the new administrator of the School of Nursing. Edna Fritz will bring to Minnesota the kind of energy and purposefulness with which it has long been familiar in her predecessor. She has earned B.S. and M.A. degrees and has all but completed work for a doctoral degree at Teachers College, Columbia. She has had the most active professional experience as head of medical and surgical nursing at the Cornell University — New York Hospital School of Nursing; she has taught basic nursing at Boston University; and for several years served the National League for Nursing in its Department of Basic and Higher Degree Programs. It was her particular assignment there to visit collegiate schools, conducting workshops and studying qualifications for accreditation. In the course of these experiences she has gained wide acquaintance within the profession. This is a major asset to an executive of a school who must be an experienced "fisher of men" (or women) if faculties are to be kept strong.

The curtain rises on the second fifty years of the School of Nursing in an atmosphere of high excitement. Leaders of the profession expect the future to be crowded with effort. The nurse of today is not concerned exclusively with the work of the parish. Nor are her ambitions bounded by the limits of the city, the state or even the nation. The international phase has begun in the history of nursing as it has begun in every other serious interest of human life.

"The price we pay for being human beings," Katharine Densford once observed, "is that we must be aware of others." The circumstances in which these simple, moving words were spoken are themselves significant. Miss Densford was talking not to a group of faculty members and students on the Minnesota campus but before a congress of Brazilian nurses assembled, in December, 1950, at San Salvador.

The day of the community nurse is by no means gone. She no longer carries, as badge of servitude, a scuffed portmanteau, crowded with odds and ends of homely remedies, but she is ever present in the person of the modern R.N., a familiar, gratefully welcomed figure in hospital and home. What is different today is that the R.N. has a colleague who sits in international conferences, is entrusted with the work of disseminating the benefits of discovery in medicine, herself contributes to the lore of the healing sciences.

The nurse has emerged from the twilight world of undefined responsibilities. She has put off the limitations with which tradition bound her so long. Today the affairs which are properly hers she conducts with authority as well as with pride and zeal. She conducts them on a world basis. The exchange of ideas, of teachers, of techniques, of all the healthy, unhesitant commitments of the world of thought are made in the belief that science must strive to establish awareness of others as a golden rule for the globe.

Because she holds this conviction securely the nurse hopes to share, during the next fifty years, in improvements of her work which will be as dramatic and rewarding as those of the past fifty years have been.

She could ask for no better destiny.

CHRONOLOGY AND INDEX

Chronology

1905–1908. Dr. Richard Olding Beard used every public forum available to him to urge the necessity of elevating the education of the nurse to the professional level in a university school.

1908, October 1. The board of regents of the University of Minnesota authorized the establishment of the first university school of nursing, the School for Nurses. Bertha Erdmann tentatively appointed superintendent of nurses and sent to Teachers College, Columbia, for further preparation.

1909, March 1. The school opened with a three-year undergraduate program in which 4 students were enrolled.

1910, July 1. The resignation of Bertha Erdmann became effective. Louise Powell named as her successor. September 1. Miss Powell took up her duties. Dr. L. B. Baldwin established as superintendent of the university hospital. September 5. Elliot Hospital opened. First clinical experience offered nurse students.

1911, February. Affiliating students from other schools of nursing accepted for the first time.

1912, June. First class, numbering 12, graduated.

1914, September. Enrollment reached 32.

1915, September. Elizabeth Pierce appointed first full-time instructor.

1916, July 1. Marion L. Vannier appointed to act as superintendent of nurses during six months' leave for Miss Powell. First course in sociology offered to nurse students.

1917, April 6. Congress declared war on Imperial German government. September. Enrollment reached 69. First affiliation with Glen Lake Sanitorium for tuberculosis nursing experience. December 13. Base Hospital Unit 26 went on active duty. With it were 65 women from Minnesota. Miss Powell acting as superintendent of the university hospital during the absence of Dr. Baldwin on war assignment in Washington. Elizabeth Pierce returned to assist during wartime emergency. Navy corpsmen began special nursing preparation under Miss Powell, Miss Vannier, and Miss Pierce.

1918, September. Flu epidemic began. November 11. Armistice signed. First course in public health nursing offered in cooperation with the Public Health Association.

1919, June. The five-year program established, leading to the degree bachelor of science and the diploma of graduate in nursing. The Self-Government Association organized.

1920, April 14. Name changed to the School of Nursing.

EDUCATION FOR NURSING

1921, February 26. An agreement reached between directors of Twin City hospitals and the university for the establishment of the Central School. March. The board of regents authorized the creation of the Central School utilizing for purpose of clinical experience the facilities of the Minneapolis General Hospital, the Charles T. Miller Hospital of St. Paul, and the Northern Pacific Beneficial Association Hospital of St. Paul. June. The official bulletin of the university carried first announcement of the establishment of the Central School.

1922, January 1. Miss Powell on leave; Miss Vannier again acting superintendent of nurses. Board of regents authorized a separate division in public health teaching. September. A course for the preparation of instructors in schools of nursing — designed in collaboration with the College of Education — added to the curriculum. Courses in public health nursing created by Anna Jones (Mariette) and Alma Haupt, members of the school's class of 1919.

1923, January 1. Miss Powell returned to assume new title as director of the school. Headquarters moved from the hospital to Millard Hall.

1924, July 1. Miss Vannier succeeded Miss Powell as director. July. Eula Butzerin assumed charge of public health nursing courses. 1924–1925. Recurrent smallpox epidemics taxed the facilities of the university hospital and the womanpower of the School of Nursing.

1926. The report of Professor Abbie Turner of Mount Holyoke to the Rockefeller Foundation said that "the work done by the School of Nursing at Minnesota easily won first place."

1927. Barbara Thompson (Sharpless), class of 1913, acting director during Miss Vannier's sabbatical leave. July. First summer school courses offered; the subjects: Administration in Schools of Nursing and Ward Teaching and Supervision.

1929. Thorough revision of the five-year curriculum by a committee consisting of Dean E. P. Lyon, medical school; Dean Melvin Haggerty, College of Education; Dr. Harold Diehl, School of Public Health; Miss Butzerin; and Miss Vannier. A new program offered leading to degree of bachelor of science conferred by the College of Education, along with the diploma, graduate in nursing. Lucile Petry (Leone) joined the faculty.

1930, July 7. Katharine J. Densford (Dreves) became director.

1931, September. Graduate curriculums in various clinical fields established. First clinical (ward) instructor in nursing history appointed: Myrtle Hodgkins (Coe).

1933, January 1. Central School discontinued. October. Enrollment 471. Dedication of Powell Hall, dormitory for nurse students.

1937, April. A psychopathic unit opened in the university hospital offering opportunity for instruction in psychiatric nursing. July. Miss Densford on sabbatical leave; Lucile Petry acting director. Miss Densford attended the International Council of Nurses at London.

1938, July. Miss Densford returned. Decision made to admit students to the three-year program in nursing only in the fall while candidates for the B.S. degree were admitted in both fall and spring. The change looked toward the gradual elimination of the three-year program.

1939, October. Ruth Harrington joined the faculty.

1940, August 27. The University accepted sponsorship of the Base Hospital Unit 26, United States Army. Public Law 146 re-enacted. Lucile Petry on leave as special consultant to the United States Public Health Service under the direction of Surgeon General Thomas Parran. Pearl McIver, class of 1919, serving as senior public health consultant. Alma Haupt, class of 1919, secretary of the advisory council on nursing service for the Red Cross. Total enrollment in the School of Nursing reached 750. Lanham Act passed. Federal aid for nursing education made available through the Smith-Hughes and George-Deen Acts.

1941, December 7. Japanese attack Pearl Harbor. June. First direct federal appropriation for nursing education made by the Congress.

CHRONOLOGY

1942. Special adjustments to wartime emergency included the admission of an additional class of three-year students and the design of a special course for college graduates, enabling them to become nurses in a two-and-a-half-year program.

1943, June 15. Bolton Bill, creating the United States Cadet Nurse Corps, signed into law by President Roosevelt. Lucile Petry resigned from the faculty of the school while on leave to become director of the Corps. July 1. The Corps came into active existence. Summer. The school conducted a pilot experiment in rural nursing education. November. The accomplishments on behalf of the Corps within the School of Nursing at Minnesota received the special commendation of the Surgeon General.

1944. Enrollment reached the thousand mark. May 15. The first induction ceremonies introducing cadet nurses to active service held on the campus. The school, at the instigation of the American Psychiatric Association, conducted experiments in advanced psychiatric nursing.

1945, May 12. Second induction ceremonies held. An addition to Powell Hall finished with Lanham funds.

1947, July 12. The three-year basic program discontinued. An experiment in practical nursing instruction begun in cooperation with the General College.

1948. The W. K. Kellogg Foundation made appropriations for the support of experimental projects in education. The formulation of a completely new plan for graduate nurse education was inaugurated. October. The rural nursing program went into full effect.

1949, October. A six-quarter course in home management and practical nursing operated jointly by the School of Nursing and the School of Agriculture launched. A full revision of the basic professional nursing curriculum resulted in the inauguration of the sixteen-quarter course.

1950, October. A program in nursing education leading to the master of education degree was begun; first degree earned, 1951.

1951, October. A program in nursing administration leading to the master of nursing administration degree begun; first degrees awarded in 1952. Opening of the Variety Club Heart Hospital offered new opportunities for study of both children and adults.

1952. A pediatric unit opened with funds provided by the Minnesota legislature.

1954. The School of Nursing participated in the work of rehabilitating educational facilities in Korea. Its efforts were directed toward modernizing instruction and equipment in the school of nursing at Seoul National University.

1955, Spring. First students in the program in nursing administration leading to the bachelor of nursing administration degree admitted; first degrees awarded in 1956.

1956. The Health Amendments Act of the Congress provided support for preparation of nurse educators and administrators assigned 33 traineeships to the School of Nursing at Minnesota.

1958, October 16. The University of Minnesota School of Nursing Foundation established.

1959. Fiftieth anniversary celebration. Retirement of Katharine Densford. Appointment of Edna Fritz as her successor.

Index